Exercises for the Jaw to Shoulder

Dr. Brian James Abelson, DC, ART
Kamali T. Abelson, B.Sc.

Kinetic Health
Calgary, Alberta, Canada

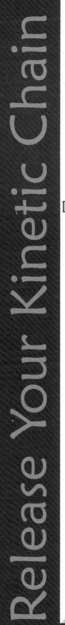

Release Your Kinetic Chain

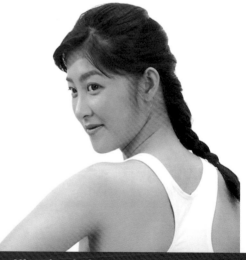

**Kinetic chain exercises for the
Release Your Body
series of books**

Canadian Cataloguing in Publication Data
Abelson, Brian and Abelson, Kamali
Exercises for the Jaw to Shoulder - Volume 1 of Release Your Kinetic Chain ©
Includes index and table of contents.

Copyright Registration	1071555
ISBN-13 - Hardcopy	978-0-9733848-4-0
ISBN-13 - E-Copy	978-0-9733848-5-7

First Printing: 2010, Rowan Tree Books Ltd.
Printed in USA 10 9 8 7 6 5 4 3 2 1

Notice: Although the authors, editors, and publishers have made every effort to ensure the accuracy and completeness of information contained in this book, it is difficult to ensure that all of the information is accurate, and the possibility of error can never be completely eliminated. The authors, editors, and publishers disclaim any liability or responsibility for injury or damage to persons or property, that is incurred as a consequence, directly or indirectly, of the use and application of any of the contents of this book, as well as for any unintentional slights to any person or entity.

Credits
Production and Editing: Kamali Abelson, Hannah MacLeod
Technical Edits: Dr. Brian J. Abelson, Dr. Tarveen Ahluhwalia
Illustrations: Lavanya Balasubramanian, 123RF Limited
Cover artwork by: Studio Sun

Certain images and/or photos in this book are the copyrighted property of 123RF Limited, its Contributors or Licensed Partners and are being used with permission under license. These images and/or photos may not be copied or downloaded without permission from 123RF Limited.

The Publishers have made every effort to trace the copyright holders for borrowed materials. If they have inadvertently overlooked any, they will be pleased to make the necessary arrangements at the first opportunity.

Kinetic Health books are available at a special discount for bulk purchase by practitioners, corporations, institutions, and other organizations. For details, see our website or contact the Special Sales Manager at Kinetic Health.

Kinetic Health® **Websites**
www.releaseyourbody.com
www.drabelson.com
www.activerelease.ca
www.youtube.com/kinetichealthonline

Canada: **Kinetic Health**
Edgemont Chiropractic – Soft Tissue Management Systems
#10 - 34 Edgedale Drive N.W.
Calgary, AB, Canada, T3A 2R4
403-241-3772 (bus)
403-241-3846 (fax)

Health Disclaimer

This book provides information about wellness management in an informational and educational manner only, with information that is general in nature and that is not specific to you, the reader. The contents of this book are intended to assist you and other readers in your personal wellness efforts.

Nothing in this book should be construed as personal advice or diagnosis, and must *not* be used in this manner. The information provided about conditions is general in nature. This information does not cover all possible uses, actions, precautions, side-effects, or interactions of medicines, or medical procedures. The information in this book should not be considered as complete and does *not* cover all diseases, ailments, physical conditions, or their treatment.

You should consult with your physician before beginning any exercise, weight loss, or health care program. This book should *not* be used in place of a call or visit to a competent health-care professional. You should consult a health care professional before adopting any of the suggestions in this book or before drawing inferences from it. Any decision regarding treatment and medication for your condition should be made with the advice and consultation of a qualified health care professional. If you have, or suspect you have, a health-care problem, then you should immediately contact a qualified health care professional for treatment.

Exercise Disclaimer

See "Exercise Disclaimer...Please read!"on page vii for details.

No Warranties

The authors, publishers, and/or their respective directors, shareholders, officers, employees, agents, trainers, contractors, representatives, or successors do not guarantee or warrant the quality, accuracy, completeness, timeliness, appropriateness or suitability of the information in this book, or of any product or services referenced by this book. The information in this book is provided on an "as is" basis and the authors and publishers make no representations or warranties of any kind with respect to this information. This book may contain inaccuracies, typographical errors, or other errors.

Liability Disclaimer

The publishers, authors, and any other parties involved in the creation, production, provision of information, or delivery of this book specifically disclaim any responsibility, and shall not be liable for any damages, claims, injuries, losses, liabilities, costs, or obligations, including any direct, indirect, special, incidental, or consequential damages (collectively known as "Damages") whatsoever and howsoever caused, arising out of, or in connection with, the use or misuse of the book and the information contained within it, whether such Damages arise in contract, tort, negligence, equity, statute law, or by way of any other legal theory.

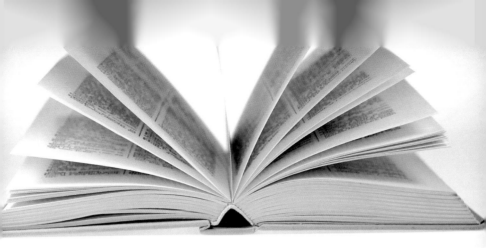

Table of Contents

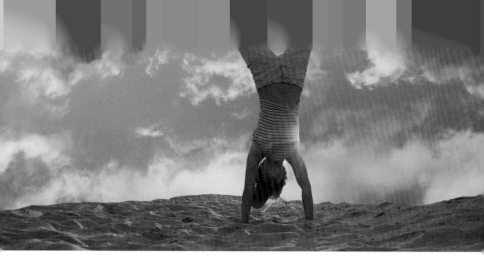

Exercise Disclaimer...Please read!

Exercise is not without its risks, and this or any other exercise program may result in injury. Risks include but are not limited to: aggravation of a pre-existing condition, risk of injury, or adverse effects of over-exertion such as muscle strain, abnormal blood pressure, fainting, disorders of heartbeat, and in very rare instances, of heart attack.

The instruction and advice presented here are in no way intended as a substitute for medical consultation. The authors and publisher disclaim any liability from and in connection with this program.

The exercises in this book are provided for educational purposes only, and are not to be interpreted as a recommendation for a specific treatment plan, product, or course of action, or as a substitute for professional supervision or advice. To reduce the risk of injury in your case, consult your doctor before beginning this or any exercise program.

The authors, publishers, and technical experts use reasonable effort to include accurate and up-to-date information in its information sources; however, all information appearing is general in nature. Kinetic Health, the authors, publishers, and practitioners do not assume liability or give any warranty of any kind for the information and data contained or omitted from this document or for any action or inaction made in reliance thereon. Information presented in this book and associated web sites may be changed at any time. Specific advice should be obtained in respect of specific situations.

Any programs involving weights, intense workouts and apparatus may put strong physical demands on any child who is still growing – supervision is obligatory in such cases. If you have or have had asthma, growth condition,

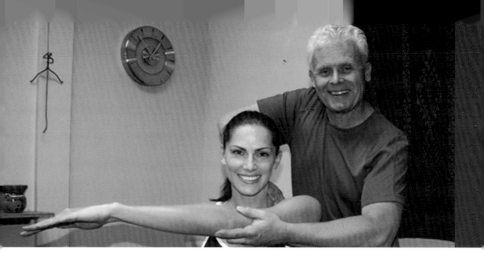

Foreword by Dr. Brian Abelson

All too often, we find our patients and athletes jumping into the advanced, intensive stages of exercise before establishing needed ground work. This rushed approach leads to more injuries and an accompanying lack of performance.

The *Release Your Kinetic Chain* series of exercise books takes a **functional** approach to exercise. With this approach, we give you step-by-step recommendations to help you move through the **rehabilitation phase** of an exercise program to prepare you for the **performance phase**.

This book (and its sister books) have two basic objectives:

- The first objective is to help you rehabilitate your body after an injury (or long period of inactivity) and prepare it for more intensive exercise programs.

- The second objective is to help you prepare your body so that it is ready for sport or athletic performance training.

Rehabilitating an Injury...do this first!

There are some basic concepts that you need to understand in order to be successful with our program. First of all, when you are rehabilitating an injury, we will always have you work in a completely **pain-free zone**. That's right...at this phase, the concept of *no pain, no gain* is completely wrong! Our primary objective with rehabilitation is to increase muscular endurance and neurological motor control. With rehabilitation routines, we always work within a pain-free zone...essentially a zone of safety where you can bring your injured areas back to normal activity.

Our family of exercise books focuses on exercise routines that help you to rehabilitate your body from previous injuries, and bring it up to speed for the next phase of performance training. Your injury could be as minor as an ankle sprain, or more substantial such as recovery from a surgery! In all cases, it is critical that you take your body through the rehabilitative exercise phase before jumping into the performance phase!

You will find that the Beginner and Intermediate routines expect you to work within this pain-free rehabilitative zone. The Advanced routines will help to transition you into the Performance or Athletic arenas.

Increasing Your Performance...wait to do this!

Only **after** you have established good muscle endurance and motor control (neurological control) should you focus upon increasing your strength or speed.

Increasing strength should only come after good neuromuscular endurance has been established. If you try to increase strength too quickly, you will discover that you have found the best formula for **developing ongoing injuries**.

In this book, we provide proven exercise routines that gradually build your strength and endurance to the point where you will be ready to begin performance training.

Why you need these books

The training programs in these books are very different from the body-building type of programs you will find in most gyms. The purpose of most body-building programs is to increase the *size* of individual body parts – that is, to develop a state of muscle hypertrophy. Body-building often trains the body, not as a set of linked kinetic chains, but as a series of unconnected segments.

This type of training can be a major mistake when you are trying to rehabilitate an injury or when you are trying to improve your sports performance. Often these body-building programs create muscle imbalances, cause even more injuries in unprepared tissues, and result in an overall decrease in performance. This is a huge price to pay, even if your initial goal was to simply increase muscle size by isolating and growing specific muscle groups.

Instead, the exercise programs in the *Release Your Kinetic Chain* book series use step-by-step procedures which take into consideration kinetic chain relationships, tissue interactions, core imbalances, elastic power, and aerobic training. We strive to give you a balanced means of achieving a good strong body that is injury-free.

■   Our exercise routines always take into consideration a key fundamental aspect of good rehabilitation – **Kinetic Chain Relationships**.   Since injury or weakness in one area of your body always affects the function of numerous other related areas, we ensure that our routines take into account direct muscular connections, muscle antagonists, fascial connections, as well as the fact that tissue restrictions affect the primary mechanisms of energy storage and release. See *"Understanding Your Kinetic Chain" on page 17.*

■   Our exercise routines always consider how the core of your body acts as the power generator for your entire body. This is true even for movements of your neck, shoulders, arms, hands, legs or feet. No matter what the action, you need a strong stable core to be able to transfer energy to your extremities. *See "Involving Your Core" on page 13.*

■   Our exercise routines also address the development of your elastic power or the ability of your muscles, ligaments, tendons, and fascia to store and release energy. The ability of your soft tissues to store and release energy is dependent upon the quality of your soft tissues. Low-quality tissues are full of adhesions, scar tissues, and knots. These tissues do not store or release energy efficiently. High-quality tissues can move easily through their full range of motion, are not restricted or adhesed, are capable of long periods of endurance, and are not easily injured. One of the primary goals of our exercise routines is to provide you with a means for improving your overall tissue quality. See *"Principle 2: Good Tissue Quality = Good Performance"* on page 9.

- Aerobic warm-ups are an integral component of all of our programs. It doesn't matter if we are dealing with a jaw, neck, shoulder, back, or leg injury; aerobic training is essential. By developing your aerobic system you increase your circulatory function and your ability to produce energy on demand. Aerobic exercise does this by increasing the density of capillaries in your muscles, and the density of mitochondria (your personal energy factories) in your cells. See *"Benefits of Cardiovascular Exercises"* on page 40.

- And finally, one of our primary goals is to give you effective strategies for increasing strength without further injuring yourself. The exercise routines we provide in these books are similar to ones that we provide to our patients. These routines have been successfully tested and improved over time, and will help you to strengthen your body in a gentle and progressive manner.

I hope you stick to the routines, enjoy this book, and benefit from your improved health. I am sure you will achieve great results.

All the best in health!

Dr. Brian Abelson

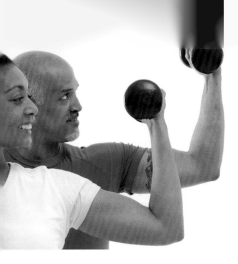

Rehabilitation vs. Athletic Training

A Kinetic Chain Perspective

Exercise protocols and training methods should be quite different when you are rehabilitating an injury to bring your body up to a functional level of activity vs. when you are striving to improve athletic performance on an already well-trained, uninjured body. After all, the goals and capabilities of the trainee are quite different within the two levels of training.

Unfortunately, most standard exercise programs do not differentiate between the two goals, and tend to apply the same exercise routines in both situations. Moving too fast, with an unprepared body, into athletic or performance training is a sure recipe for injury and disaster.

The objective of our *Release Your Kinetic Chain* series of exercise books is to provide exercises that help you resolve injuries in specific areas of your body, and that prepare your body for the more difficult performance-based workouts. These books provide a step-by-step, methodical process, that requires patience, and time on your part.

Let's take a few minutes to understand the difference between these two types of programs – *Rehabilitative* and *Athletic* Training.

About Rehabilitative Exercise Routines

Rehabilitation programs focus upon returning your body to a state of full function without further injuring yourself in the process. Our primary objective with our rehabilitation programs is to resolve your injury, increase neurological and motor control, build strength, and increase flexibility while restoring function.

Only after you have rehabilitated completely from an injury, and have restored good muscle endurance and motor control (neurological control) should you consider applying athletic performance strategies to your training.

Rehabilitation training is not just for resolving existing injuries, it is also a critical preliminary step for preparing your body to accept and benefit from advanced conditioning and performance training. If you have not been physically active for a period of time, it is essential that you start with the *Beginner* sections of this book. As you work your way through the exercise levels, you will be tuning and preparing your body for more advanced performance-based exercises.

Rehabilitaton requires patience and time! Remember, your body needs time to heal from your injuries. Many people, in their enthusiasm to reach their goal, make their injuries worse by not giving their body sufficient time to heal. So take the time to properly prepare your body for athletic level training.

What we provide in these books are guidelines for gently tuning your body without causing undue stress, injury, or pain! But it is your responsibility to *listen to your body, understand its signals,* and adjust your routines accordingly.

The following rules are a few fundamental principles that you should keep in mind as you work through your rehabilitative routines:

- ■ *Principle 1: No Pain...All Gain! - page 3.*
- ■ *Principle 2: Develop your Power - page 4.*
- ■ *Principle 3: Build your Aerobic Base - page 6.*

Principle I: No Pain...All Gain!

Rehabilitation (unlike athletic training) requires that you perform your exercises within a *completely pain-free* zone; essentially a *zone of safety.*

Exercising in a manner that causes pain develops abnormal neuromuscular patterns that may lead to further injury. Conventional rehabilitation strategies commonly do not succeed because they do not address the underlying neuromuscular problems. They are often designed to make you work through your pain (as in work-hardening programs). This only causes you to create or reinforce the abnormal motor responses which in turn continues to keep you in pain.

In addition, if you work through pain caused by tissue damage you run the risk of *central sensitization.* This is a nervous system process which causes you to become more sensitive to pain. The only way to break this pattern is to perform your exercises in a pain-free zone.

We commonly have patients come to our clinic who have exercised through their pain for years! They are always amazed at how, by exercising within a pain-free zone, we were able to help them break their pain-cycle in just a few short weeks.

What works will vary from person to person so *listen to your body* and adjust the routines accordingly.

Bottom line:

Never work through injury pain.

If you have an injury, and the exercise hurts during certain motions, or if you feel pain when resting, then restrict the range of motion of the exercise to lie within your pain-free range.

In addition, avoid the exercises that currently cause you pain, until your body is ready for them.

To truly rehabilitate your injuries, you must work within a **pain-free** zone.

This is quite different from training to improve your performance where you may have to endure some degree of muscle pain (not injury pain) to improve strength and endurance.

Principle 2: Develop your Power

Power (within your body) is about the production and transfer of force through your entire body. Power is also a function of how well you can recruit your nervous system to control muscular action. The more efficient your nervous system, the more power you will have. The more power you have, the easier it is to perform your activities and exercises without injury.

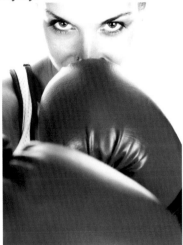

Power is not the same as strength; power is about maximum efficiency without effort. (Strength requires a lot of effort and energy.)

The more power you have, the less energy you will need to expend to perform a task, which equates to having more energy available to heal and grow your body.

Power generation is also directly related to the **quality** of your soft tissues (muscles, ligaments, tendons, etc.). The quality of your soft tissues determine how well you can store and release energy.

Think of your soft tissues as being like cords of elastic rubber (or perhaps a telephone cord). Just like a rubber cord you can stretch (storing energy) and contract them (releasing energy). In a healthy state, your muscles contract and release instantaneously, storing and releasing energy with changes in body motion.

So what happens when a rubber cord gets knots tied in it? The rubber cord's ability to store and release energy is immediately diminished. The same thing happens to your soft tissues when you build up restrictions and adhesions (from the micro-tears caused by repetitive motion), or scar tissue from injuries. These adhesions and scar tissues are analogous to knots in the cord. Just as the cord's ability to store and release energy was diminished by knots, so is our body's ability to store and release energy diminished by these restrictions. Think of these adhesions and restrictions as *energy leaks* that rob your body of much needed energy for healing.

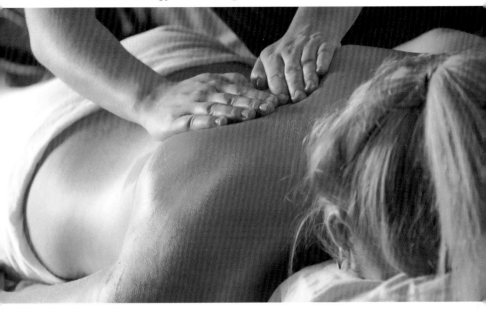

You will have problems with storing and releasing your own energy if your body is full of tight areas and ropy fibrous restrictions. This is why foam rollers, Massage Therapy, Active Release Techniques, Graston Techniques, and dozens of other soft tissue techniques are so valuable for helping in your healing process. All these procedures act to improve the quality of your soft tissue by releasing or removing the soft tissue restrictions that lie between your tissue layers.

Bottom line, you may need to invest in some soft tissue care to get rid of these restrictions...these restrictions are sapping your energy, causing injuries, and aging you prematurely. Consider getting treatment for these areas. Obtaining care in this area is an investment that will pay countless positive dividends to you for the rest of your life.

Principle 3: Build your Aerobic Base

Yes, rehabilitative care does require you to build a good aerobic base. Your cardiovascular system is responsible for transporting oxygen and nutrients to all your cells, and for carrying away toxins and waste products.

These are essential processes for any kind of recovery from injuries, and even more essential if you plan to take up athletic endeavours. See the following topics for more information about the importance of Aerobic warm-ups:

- *Benefits of Cardiovascular Exercises - page 40*
- *So what is a good warm-up? - page 43*
- *Working within your Aerobic Zone - page 44*

Athletic or Performance Care Routines

The *Release Your Kinetic Chain* series of books focuses on helping you resolve your injuries and preparing your body for performance level training.

- If your primary objective is to resolve an injury and you have no interest in athletic or performance care, then you can move directly to the next chapter.

- For the rest of you, there are several factors you should consider once you have attained a level of fitness where your body is ready to begin performance training.

Athletic performance training is all about speed, power, and strength, which in turn are based on the development of superb neuromuscular control. Great neuromuscular control (the training of your nervous system to perform a task) is what defines the world's best athletes – not strength or muscle size. There are some similarities (as well as some huge differences) in the objectives of rehabilitative exercise and athletic or performance training. In both, the development of neuromuscular control remains critical.

Athletic or Performance training has greater risks than rehabilitation training. Athletic training often involves riding the fence between overloading the body (to increase strength and power) and reaching the point of tissue failure (injury). With Performance training, there is always a greater chance of injury.

Athletic or Performance training differs from rehabilitative training in its:

- Increased risk of injury.
- Need to work through muscle pain.
- Need to increase resistance to the point of overloading the muscles.
- Requiring speed training.
- Development of the anaerobic system.

Before Beginning Athletic Training

The following are a few fundamental principles that you should keep in mind before you start the Athletic or Performance training routines:

- *Principle 1: Athletic Development is Not the Same as Body-Building! - page 8*
- *Principle 2: Good Tissue Quality = Good Performance - page 9*
- *Principle 3: Some Muscle Pain is Okay - page 10*
- *Principle 4: Develop Your Aerobic Zone Before Working on Your Anaerobic Zone - page 11*

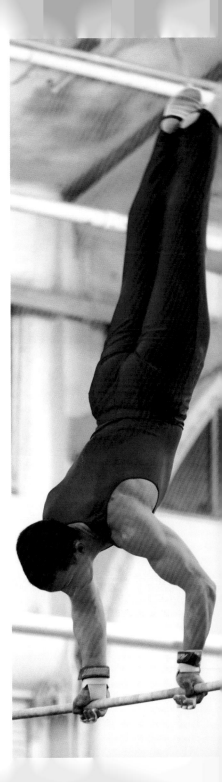

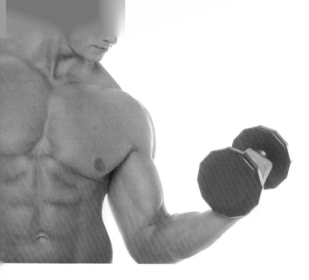

Principle 1: Athletic Development is Not the Same as Body-Building!

Exercise programs that focus only on increasing muscle size serve to meet *body-building* objectives of increasing size and definition and have very little to do with improved athletic performance or improved body function.

Athletic Performance training typically focuses upon developing your speed, power, and strength. To achieve this goal, you must establish good muscle endurance, good motor control, and superb neuromuscular responses. This is very different from body-building which focuses primarily on increasing the size and bulk of your muscles.

Exercise programs that focus only on increasing muscle size by isolating specific muscles (weight training with machines) often result in muscular imbalances, soft tissue injuries, and an overall decrease in performance. This is one of the reasons we do not recommend the use of exercise machines (other than cable machines) in any of our routines.

Look for athletic training programs that integrate elements of strength, endurance, speed, and power. These are the ones that will be most helpful in increasing your performance.

Principle 2: Good Tissue Quality = Good Performance

In sports performance, the quality of your soft tissue is a key element that cannot be ignored. When you improve the quality of your tissue (no restrictions, adhesions, or tightness) then you will reap the rewards of faster recovery, increased speed, improved range of motion, more strength, reduced injuries, and improved performance.

As we discussed in *Principle 2: Develop your Power - page 4*, your muscles are like rubber bands. When there are no knots (restrictions) in them you can easily store and release your energy. This directly translates into improved performance. This is why soft tissue techniques such as Active Release Techniques have helped take Olympic athletes to gold medal status. These types of techniques improve the overall quality of your soft tissues.

Bottom line: When you ignore the quality and state of your soft tissues, then you are taking the path of diminished performance! So, if you have restrictions and tight spots that are not resolved by exercising, then take the time to work these restrictions out by using our myofascial techniques (foam rollers, tennis balls, self-massage) or see a skilled soft tissue practitioner for help in restoring your soft tissue quality. See *Alternative Therapies to Explore - page 195* for more information.

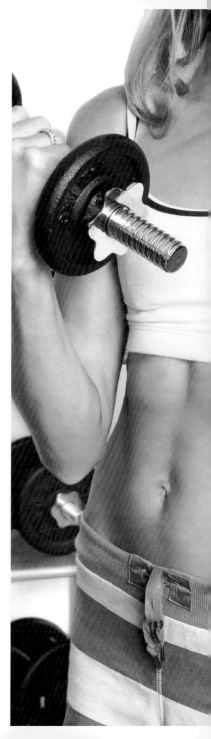

Principle 3: Some Muscle Pain is Okay

With performance training, it is often necessary to work through your muscle pain.

I am often asked the question, *"How do I know the difference between acceptable muscle pain and injury pain?"*

Muscle pain from exercising will usually diminish with time, but pain from an injury will not. I tell my patients that they should never work an area if they feel constant pain even when they are *not* exercising.

Pain from an injury is usually quite distinctive with sharp, stabbing sensations – or much more intense than normal muscle pain. It is also common to have injury- related pain increase with physical activity.

If you are injured, you need to return to a rehabilitative approach in your exercise program (for the affected structure). Working through injury-related pain is a sure way of continuing the injury or creating even more severe problems.

Principle 4: Develop Your Aerobic Zone Before Working on Your Anaerobic Zone

Anaerobic training (where your tissues are working with reduced oxygen levels) is an essential aspect of performance training. However, as we mentioned earlier, you must first establish a good aerobic base before you can even consider beginning your anaerobic training.

Athletes who fail to train their aerobic base to a sufficient level before embarking on anaerobic training (intervals) can find themselves dealing with soft tissue injuries, diminished energy, slow healing, and even decreased performance levels. See *Working within your Aerobic Zone - page 44* for more details about aerobic training.

The anaerobic or lactate system is very different from your aerobic system since it only operates for 5 seconds to about 2 minutes. This anaerobic system is very efficient at producing power, but it also produces a considerable amount of waste by-products.

Do not start anaerobic training until you have established and maintained your *aerobic base* for several months. Once you start anaerobic training, your *Lactate Threshold* is established as you move back and forth between your aerobic and anaerobic systems. Your goal is to increase your anaerobic capacity (Lactate Threshold) since this will allow you to train for longer periods of time (within your aerobic zone), at faster speeds, and with greater intensity. A higher Lactate Threshold will also allow you to recover faster from your workouts.

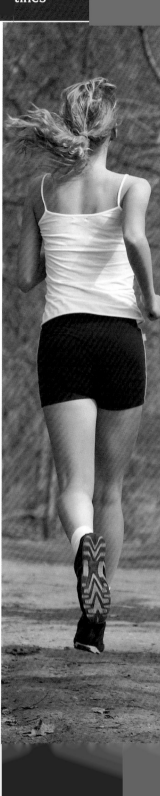

Comparing the Benefits of Aerobic and Anaerobic Training

Cardiovascular warm-ups are all about increasing your circulatory function and increasing your energy production. Building up your aerobic base makes you heal faster, perform better, and even turns back your biological clock! Aerobic exercise does this by:

- Increasing the density of capillaries in your muscles.

- Increasing the mitochondrial function of your cells

Serious anaerobic training should only be taken up after you have built a good aerobic base. Anaerobic training causes your body to increase its production of Human Growth Hormone, which brings a whole host of health benefits to your body.

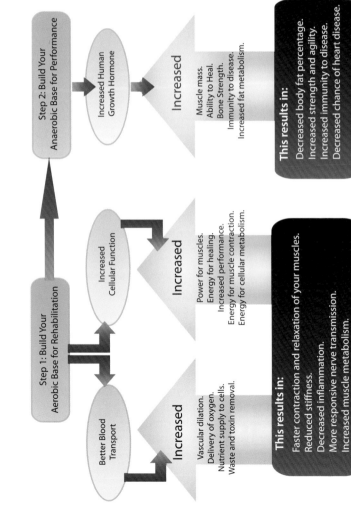

Step 1: Build Your Aerobic Base for Rehabilitation

Step 2: Build Your Anaerobic Base for Performance

Better Blood Transport

Increased Cellular Function

Increased Human Growth Hormone

Increased

Vascular dilation.
Delivery of oxygen.
Nutrient supply to cells.
Waste and toxin removal.

Increased

Power for muscles.
Energy for healing.
Increased performance.
Energy for muscle contraction.
Energy for cellular metabolism.

Increased

Muscle mass.
Ability to Heal.
Bone Strength.
Immunity to disease.
Increased fat metabolism.

This results in:

Faster contraction and relaxation of your muscles.
Reduced stiffness.
Decreased inflammation.
More responsive nerve transmission.
Increased muscle metabolism.
Increased muscle function.

This results in:

Decreased body fat percentage.
Increased strength and agility.
Increased immunity to disease.
Decreased chance of heart disease.

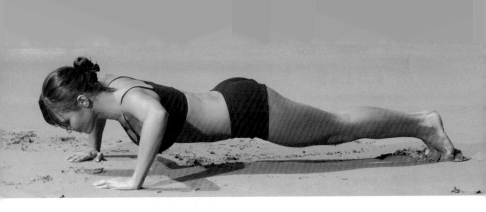

Involving Your Core

It doesn't matter what type of exercise you are performing; all exercises require good posture and solid support from your core. Your core is the foundation and source of all your movements, providing a stable base for all arm, leg, and neck motions. Your ability to maintain good posture is greatly dependent upon your core stability!

If you have a stable, balanced, elastic core, then you can easily transfer energy from the centre of your body to all your extremities! This process of first storing energy, and then releasing it, is very similar to how a spring mechanism works. A compressed spring contains stored energy. When the spring releases, the stored energy is released to allow the spring to expand. The muscles of your core act like a spring, compressing or tightening to store energy, and expanding to release the stored energy for use in movement!

Having the ability to store and release energy from your core is a fundamental aspect of injury resolution and athletic performance. It does not matter how fit you currently are, what your age is, or what your current health status is...you can always improve the quality of your core.

If you do not have a strong core, you rob yourself of much needed power and energy, and make yourself more susceptible to injuries.

Bracing Your Core

Almost all of our exercises require you to activate, brace, and otherwise involve your core! One of the key ways that all exercises can be converted into *core* exercises is through the process of **bracing**. I first learned about this process from Dr. Stuart McGill, Department Chair of the Spine Biomechanics Laboratory at the University of Waterloo.

Bracing refers to the process of "*contracting all the muscles in the abdominal wall without drawing or pushing in*"[1]. This is very different from the common advice given by some trainers to suck in (or hollow-out) your abdominals or to contract (pull in) your Transversus Abdominis muscle (TVA). In fact, Dr. McGill's research has shown that the action of *pulling in* your TVA actually **de-activates your paraspinal muscles** causing increased instability by creating or reinforcing abnormal neuromuscular patterns.

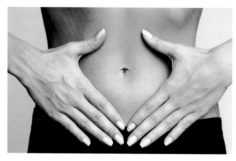

Basically, bracing is the process of gently pushing out while contracting all of your abdominal muscles.

This process also forces your paraspinal muscles to tighten at the same time.

The process of bracing creates a belt or corset around the core of your body which gives you a base of stabilization. This base of stability allows you to direct energy from your core to your extremities.

1. Ultimate Back Fitness and Performance, 3rd Edition, Stuart McGill PhD. 2004, Wabuno Publishers, BackFitPro Publishers.

How to Brace your Core!

Bracing is accomplished by gently pushing *out* your abdominal wall while tightening your back at the same time. This is actually quite a simple procedure once you get used to it. When bracing is done correctly, you will almost immediately feel like you have a stronger core.

Another way to quickly learn how to brace is by using a hula-hoop.

That's right...your childhood toy can help you brace properly, especially when you use a weighted hula-hoop. Hula-hooping forces you to brace all your abdominal and back muscles at the same time.

Many adults are surprised to discover just how difficult hooping can be initially, especially when their children find it to be so easy. This is because children generally have better core strength than their parents.

Just five minutes of hula-hooping a day can substantially increase your core stability. So pick up that hoop and have some fun!

Note: For a better understanding of your core, I recommend reading Dr. Stuart McGill's book, "**Ultimate Back Fitness and Performance**".

Understanding Your Kinetic Chain

Jaw, neck, and shoulder...what's the connection? We don't normally think of these structures as being interconnected...until we suffer from pain or injury to one of these areas. And suddenly, we become very aware of the inter-relationships between these areas. Our bodies are a remarkable series of kinetically linked systems which, when working efficiently, store and release impressive amounts of energy when we need it!

A Kinetic Chain - Jaw to Shoulder

It is important to understand that our body is one very large **Kinetic Web,** in which tension within one area directly affects the soft tissue structures in adjacent areas.

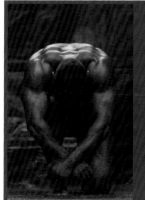

The Kinetic Web can be thought of as a linked series of kinetic chains. Each kinetic chain is made up of individual links (your joints, bones, and soft tissues) which are connected to each other to form a Kinetic Web.

Any weak link in this chain not only generates its own set of problems, but also creates problems and compensations within its entire Kinetic Web.

When a structure in your jaw, neck, or shoulder is injured or restricted, it becomes unable to effectively perform its normal functions such as chewing your food, turning your neck, or even shrugging your shoulder.

Your body compensates for this lack of ability by using other surrounding structures to help perform these actions. These compensations initially affect muscles, ligaments, tendons, and connective tissue. But as time goes on, these compensations can lead to reduced nervous system function (due to impingement upon neurological structures), reduced blood flow (cardiovascular dysfunction), and increased inflammation (due to micro-tears or biochemical changes within your body).

The bottom-line is that when you have changes in one area of your body, there will be cascading effects throughout the rest of your body, and thus throughout all the structures in your kinetic chain. These kinetic chain relationships must be taken into consideration by any soft tissue treatment or exercise protocol.

Exercise Routines and Your Kinetic Chain

Unfortunately, many exercise programs do *not* take into account the kinetic chain relationships of your body's joints, muscles, tendons, ligaments, and connective tissues.

Many exercise programs only focus on the area showing symptoms of pain and inflammation, and fail to address the structures that interconnect with these symptomatic areas. Since such programs do not address the entire kinetic chain, they are rarely effective for resolving your injury or problem.

This is why we have combined the exercises for the jaw, neck, and shoulder (and related core exercises) within one book. These three areas can often be thought of as an interwoven series of kinetic links, with each link affecting the function of the next link in the chain.

A soft tissue problem in one of these linked areas can cascade into problems in adjacent areas. It can even affect kinetic links in distant parts of your body such as your core or hips. For example a shoulder problem in a runner affects that runner's ability to transfer energy from their upper extremity through their core to their lower extremity. When this happens, your shoulder problem actually affects the **power** of your stride!

It is also important to remember that a lack of obvious symptoms (pain, inflammation) in an area does not mean that those structures have not been affected. They are still involved in performing the action, and still feel the effects of restrictions in your kinetic chain.

This is why the exercise routines in this book focus upon more than just one area. It is essential to address multiple links in your kinetic chain in order to be successful at achieving full resolution of an injury and to reach your full functional potential.

Your Jaw-to-Shoulder Kinetic Chain

The TMJ (Temporomandibular Joint) is considered to be one of the most complex joints in the human body. The TMJ works like a hinge but can also perform sliding motions.

When the TMJ and its accompanying soft tissues are restricted or unbalanced, it can result in conditions such as headaches, earaches, facial pain, vision problems, eye pain, teeth problems, balance issues, tinnitus, throat and neck pain, dizziness, and a host of other symptoms.

Most of these complaints arise from the muscles that surround the temporomandibular joint and the joint itself.

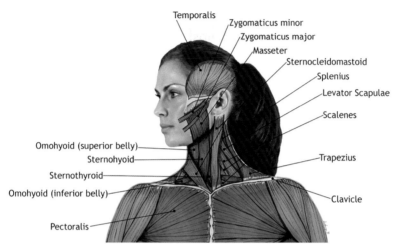

Temporalis
Zygomaticus minor
Zygomaticus major
Masseter
Sternocleidomastoid
Splenius
Levator Scapulae
Scalenes
Omohyoid (superior belly)
Sternohyoid
Sternothyroid
Omohyoid (inferior belly)
Trapezius
Pectoralis
Clavicle

Kinetic Chain components of the Jaw, Neck, and Shoulder.
Problems in any one of these areas can cause pain or dysfunction in any of the related kinetic chain structures. Remember, a lack of symptoms in an area does *not* mean that area remains unaffected.

From a kinetic chain perspective, the movements of your jaw, neck, and shoulders are directly linked. For example, the activation of the neck and jaw muscles occurs in concert with movements of the TMJ, cervical spine, and the atlanto-occipital joints.[1] (Atlanto-occipital refers to the joint that lies between the base of the skull (occiput) and the C1 vertebra (atlas)).

Thus, any injury to the neck or shoulder muscles can directly affect jaw function. Problems in one area of your kinetic chain can rapidly cascade to structures in adjacent areas. This is a key concept to keep in mind when evaluating problems with your jaw, since the source of the problem could originate from neck, shoulders, and even your core!

1. Deranged jaw–neck motor control in whiplash-associated disorders, European Journal of Oral Sciences, February, 2004; 112: 25–32. Per-Olof Eriksson, Hamayun Zafar, Birgitta Haggman-Henrikson

When you keep the inter-relationships of this kinetic chain in mind, it becomes much easier to resolve jaw problems. This is the logic we apply when prescribing exercises to our patients for the jaw, neck, and shoulder. By integrating an *appropriate* combination of jaw, neck, and shoulder exercises, we are able to achieve a greater beneficial effect for our patients.

A Case Study...Jaw to Hips!

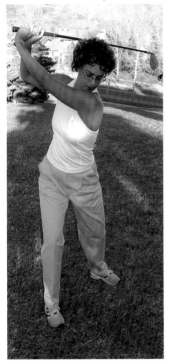

Let me give you an example about the importance of looking at all the structures of your kinetic chain. One of my patients, an ardent golfer, presented with chronic TMJ problems. She had already tried every exercise program and medical treatment that she could find, but obtained only minimal or short-lived results.

This particular patient golfed a minimum of 4 to 5 times a week, as well as during every additional spare moment that she could find.

Upon completing my physical examination, not surprisingly, I found numerous areas that needed to be addressed from her TMJ, to her neck, and shoulders. Even more interesting was discovering just how weak and unbalanced her core was.

To my patient's surprise, what started as a TMJ analysis transformed into a golf-swing analysis. On observation of her golf swing, it was easy to see that there were major restrictions in her hip which inhibited her ability to perform a full golf swing. To compensate for her restricted hip, her shoulders were forced to over-rotate, resulting in increased tension in her shoulder muscles. This tension then cascaded through her *neck* and into her *jaw*!

Previous treatments had only focused on her jaw. But, keeping in mind the kinetic chain restrictions we had identified, we chose to address all areas of restriction – from her hips, into her core, and up into the shoulders, neck, and jaw.

Although the jaw treatment techniques we used (Active Release Techniques) were very similar to those used by other practitioners, it was by combining the treatment of restricted structures throughout the jaw–neck–shoulder–core kinetic chain with appropriate exercises that gave her the result she was looking for! It wasn't long before we saw some very substantial and positive changes.

Within a few weeks of treatment and exercises, we were able to completely resolve her long-standing jaw problem. By releasing the restrictions in her *hips* and *core* we were able to resolve a long-standing problem in her *jaw*! Not only did her pain disappear, but to her delight, she was also able to realize a substantial improvement in her golf game!

Sometimes it is just that simple! In this case the weak link in her kinetic chain was her hip! By correcting that problem, we were able to also resolve problems in her shoulders, neck, and jaw!

Your Neck's Kinetic Chain

Your neck is a remarkable piece of engineering. It must be strong enough to support the weight of a small bowling ball, yet remain flexible enough to bend, flex, extend, and rotate with precision.

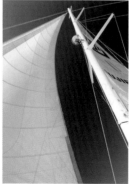

Think of your neck as a mast on a sailboat, surrounded by the rigging lines which control and stabilize the mast.

In your case, these rigging lines are made up of the muscles, tendons, ligaments, and connective tissues of your neck. These 'lines' work remarkably well as long as you maintain a fine balance of strength and flexibility.

Your neck's rigging (the lines of soft tissue that connect into your neck) make up part of your neck's kinetic chain. It is incredibly interesting to see just how far these 'lines' run, and just where many of the structures that connect into your neck insert or originate.

Your neck consists of the top seven vertebrae of your spine, the muscles and soft tissues that support and move your neck, and the blood vessels and nerves that pass from your brain to the rest of your body. A normal, healthy neck should be strong, flexible, balanced, and provide great motor control.

An understanding of this anatomical organization will give you a much better picture of your neck's kinetic chain. Consider just two of the neck's soft tissue structures:

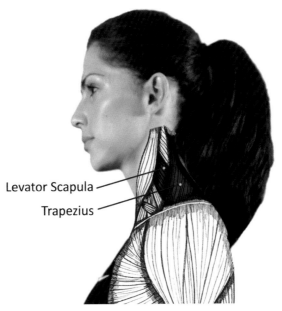

Levator Scapula
Trapezius

- **Levator Scapula Muscle:** This posterior neck muscle connects into the transverse processes of the top four vertebrae of your neck. This muscle also attaches into the top inside corner of your shoulder blade (scapula).

- **Trapezius Muscle:** This large triangular muscle inserts right at the base of your skull (occiput). However, if you follow this muscle, you will see that it also runs all the way from your mid/lower back (T12 vertebra), attaches to your shoulder blade (scapula), and extends over your shoulder to the lateral one-third of your collar bone (clavicle).

Now, consider how restrictions in any part of these structures can detrimentally affect the function of your neck. By seeing these connections, we start to understand how restrictions in distant parts of your body can affect the function and pain felt by your neck! Now let's take a look at these examples from a kinetic chain perspective:

Since the Levator Scapulae muscle connects directly into your shoulder blade, any restrictions that affects *scapular rotation* will have an immediate effect on your neck. For example, restrictions in the Serratus Anterior (which runs from your ribs to the lateral aspect of your shoulder blade) affects the function of the Levator Scapulae muscle by causing abnormal scapular rotation. This in turn increases tension in the Levator Scapulae muscle. This type of abnormal scapular motion is known as "scapular dyskinesis". Scapular dyskinesis is often a cause of chronic neck and shoulder pain.

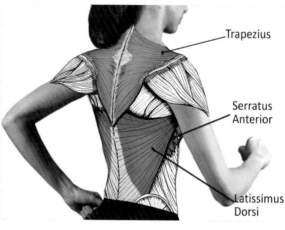

Trapezius

Serratus Anterior

Latissimus Dorsi

The Trapezius (as an adductor) and the Serratus Anterior (as an abductor) help stabilize the shoulder. The **trapezius** muscle also connects into the shoulder blade (acromion of the scapula).

Again, any abnormal motion or tension in muscles that attach to the shoulder blade will cause tension in the trapezius muscle.

Each muscle in the neck is affected not only by its adjacent structures but also by the total symmetry of all the other soft tissue structures that surround the neck.

An understanding of these key kinetic chain relationships is fundamental to injury resolution, otherwise even the best treatments and exercises will only provide symptomatic relief instead of addressing the root cause of your problems.

Neurological Impact of the Neck's Kinetic Chain

In addition to the immediate kinetic chain connections that we can see with *adjacent* soft tissue structures, we must also consider how the nervous system in the affected area of the kinetic chain directly impacts the function of the entire body.

Whenever an injury occurs in your neck (such as a sprain/strain), it damages not only the ligaments, tendons, and muscle fibres, but also their embedded neurological structures (Golgi tendon organs, muscle spindles, and joint receptors). These neurological structures play an essential role in postural control. Any damage to these structures can affect overall spinal stability, and lead to chronic back problems.

In order to get a better understanding of the importance of these neck muscles and their role in controlling body posture and gait, let us consider the suboccipital muscles (located at the base of your skull).

The suboccipital muscles (rectus capitis major and minor, superior and inferior obliques) are extremely important since they contain very high concentrations of *muscle spindle fibres.* Muscle spindles are the part of your nervous system that provide postural information to the central nervous system. Damage to these structures can result in gait disturbances and ataxia (an inability to coordinate voluntary muscle movements).

When we compare the density of muscle spindles that pass through or occupy the suboccipital area, to that of other muscles in the spine, it becomes obvious just how much this area affects whole body function.

Take a minute to review the density of muscle spindles per gram of muscle tissue:[1]

Table 1: Density of Muscle Spindles per gram of muscle tissue

Area of body	Density of spindles/ gm of muscle tissue
Inferior Oblique (Upper Neck)	242
Superior Oblique (Upper Neck)	190
Rectus Capitis Posterior Major (Upper Neck)	98
Rectus Capitis Posterior Minor (Upper Neck)	98
Longus Colli (Front of Neck)	48.6
Multifidus (Deep back muscle)	24.3
Lateral Pterygoid (Jaw muscle)	20.3
Opponens Pollicis (Hand Muscle)	17.3
Trapezius(Shoulder muscle)	2.2
Latissimus Dorsi (Large back muscle)	1.4

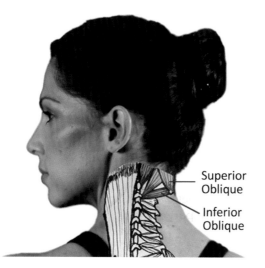

Superior Oblique

Inferior Oblique

The higher the density of muscle spindles/gm of muscle tissue, the greater the involvement of this area in maintaining whole-body postural control.

Given this, you can see that the *inferior oblique* muscle (located at the base of your skull) contains 242 spindles/gm of muscle tissue, while the very large latissimus dorsi (large back muscle) only contains 1.4 spindles/gm of muscle tissue.

Even though the inferior oblique is located at the base of your skull, due to the density of muscle spindles in this area, a restriction in this

1. Quantitative Study of Muscle Spindles in Suboccipital Muscles of Human Foetuses, Neurology India, 49, December 2001: 355-359

muscle can affect far distant structures; from your neck through to your lower back.

The key point is that any exercise program or treatment protocol must address and resolve issues within all the structures making up your neck's kinetic chain. This is required in order to deal with the consequences of restrictions which impact the neck's physical kinetic chain and cascade into your neurological control mechanisms.

This is why you need to perform *all* the exercises recommended within each routine, even when you cannot see its connection to your particular problem. We have found this method to be the most successful approach for treating our patients.

Your Shoulder's Kinetic Chain

Your shoulder's kinetic chain is made up of a complex series of related structures (links) which connect your shoulders to your neck, arms, core, hips, and lower extremities. These connections include muscles, ligaments, tendons, and connective tissues.

Your shoulder is a truly amazing piece of engineering. When functioning correctly, force and energy are easily transferred from your hips and lower extremity, through your core, and into your shoulders.

But, as remarkable as these interconnections are, they can also be the root cause of many chronic dysfunctions. That is why our exercise routines focus on key areas of power transference with a focus on whole-body stability.

As we discussed earlier, your body's kinetic chain can be viewed as a synergistic chain of links. When one part of the link goes down, the whole chain loses function.

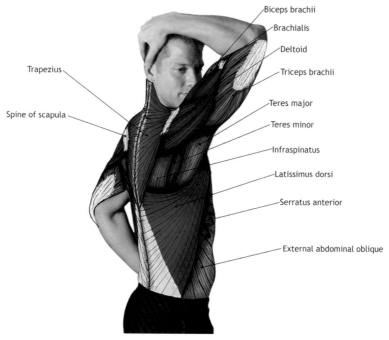

The Shoulder's Kinetic Chain

Your shoulder joint is a complex ball-and-socket joint consisting of three major osseous structures (scapula, clavicle, and humerus), as well as numerous connecting soft tissue structures (muscles, ligaments, tendons, arteries, veins, and nerves). Injury or restriction to any combination of these structures can result in restricted mobility and inability to use your shoulder.

To understand this principle as it relates to your shoulder, let us consider one of these links — the **Latissimus Dorsi** muscle.

- Normally, the latissimus dorsi functions to extend your arm, adduct your arm (bringing your arm towards the centre of your body), and internally rotate your arm at the shoulder joint.

- The latissimus dorsi originates at the crest of your pelvis (iliac crest), connects to the spinous processes of the thoracic vertebrae (T7 to T12), and inserts into your upper arm (intertubercular groove of the humerus) as part of the shoulder complex.

Because of the latissimus dorsi's numerous attachment sites, any restriction in this muscle has the potential to cause problems from the hips right up to the shoulder. Restrictions anywhere along this path can result in reduced shoulder function. Yes, we recognize that it is strange to imagine that a restriction in your hip is contributing to all those shoulder problems, but it occurs quite often.

Examine the image in *The Shoulder's Kinetic Chain - page 28* to see how all the depicted structures affect the function of your shoulder. Once you understand these kinetic chain inter-relationships, it becomes obvious why our exercise recommendations focus on much more than strengthening or stretching isolated muscle groups in just the shoulder joint.

The exercise recommendations we have given are based on the execution of functional movement patterns which increase total body motor control and integrate all the elements of your kinetic chain. These same exercise routines have delivered great results again and again at our clinic (Kinetic Health – Calgary).

So do yourself a favour, and perform *all* the exercises in each routine. Even if you don't understand the connections, trust that they are there, and carry them out! The results will be well worth your effort.

Case Study - Shoulder Kinetic Chain

One of the best ways to explain the shoulder's kinetic chain relationship, and some key therapeutic concepts, would be to introduce you to the case history of a young baseball pitcher by the name of Josh – a very talented pitcher with great potential in the game.

Josh presented to our clinic with complaints of shoulder pain with intermittent bouts of neck and jaw pain. He had a slowly progressing shoulder injury that severely affected his pitching speed and accuracy. To say the least, he was very distressed by the increasing pain and decreasing performance in his sport.

I ran Josh through the usual orthopedic and neurological tests, and found that they all showed negative (no significant findings). With hands–on palpation, I could feel muscle tension throughout the shoulders, neck, and jaw. There were no apparent signs of muscle tears, impingement syndrome, or overt muscle weakness.

We then went outside and I took a video of Josh pitching a few balls. A video analysis is a great method for obtaining biomechanical information that is not easily identified with standard tests. During the video analysis, I looked at each section frame–by–frame.

You can break down the phases of a baseball pitch into: *windup, late–cocking, acceleration*, and *follow-through*. Here is what I saw on Josh's video.

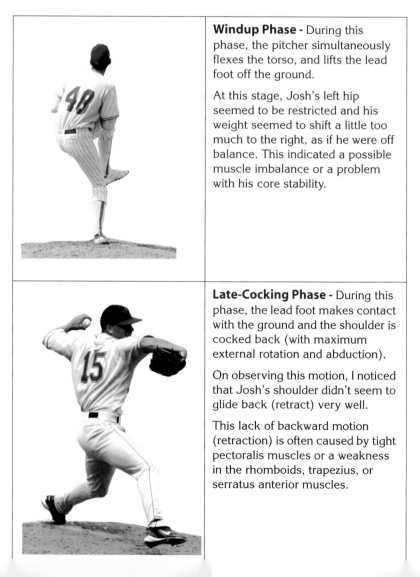

Windup Phase - During this phase, the pitcher simultaneously flexes the torso, and lifts the lead foot off the ground.

At this stage, Josh's left hip seemed to be restricted and his weight seemed to shift a little too much to the right, as if he were off balance. This indicated a possible muscle imbalance or a problem with his core stability.

Late-Cocking Phase - During this phase, the lead foot makes contact with the ground and the shoulder is cocked back (with maximum external rotation and abduction).

On observing this motion, I noticed that Josh's shoulder didn't seem to glide back (retract) very well.

This lack of backward motion (retraction) is often caused by tight pectoralis muscles or a weakness in the rhomboids, trapezius, or serratus anterior muscles.

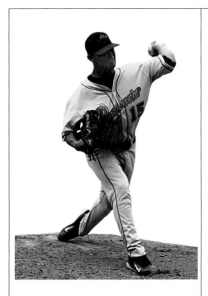

Acceleration Phase - During this phase, the shoulder must be in a stable position for maximum acceleration.

I noticed that Josh's arm seemed to move in an abnormal pattern, moving slightly out to the side.

Abnormal motion patterns (dyskinesis) are a common occurrence with chronic shoulder problems and become a matter of concern when this pattern continues for long periods of time.

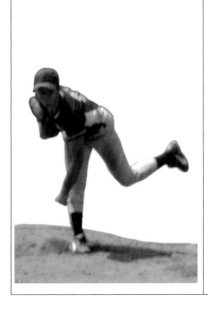

Follow Through Phase - During this phase, the ball is released, the arm internally rotates, and then is pulled in towards (adduction) the body. These actions are controlled by the trapezius, rhomboids, posterior deltoid, serratus anterior, and the teres minor muscles.

With Josh, I noticed that his upper arm (proximal humerus) seemed to move a bit too far forward (protracted) from his shoulder joint.

This is a concern since excessive forward-shoulder motion is often related to a condition known as *hyperangulation*. This condition is often linked to shoulder impingement syndromes and is common in pitchers or any sport where an overhead action is required.

This was an interesting case since a simple video analysis of Josh's shoulder problem quickly showed issues within three key kinetic chains.

- His hip and core were unstable creating abnormal compensations throughout his body.
- His restricted ability to move his shoulder back (retract) showed that he had weak posterior shoulder muscles and restricted, inflexible chest muscles.
- The hypermobility when moving the shoulder forward indicated instability in the shoulder joint.
- The developing instability in his shoulder was setting him up for a future chronic shoulder injury (impingement syndrome).

Fortunately Josh's case was quite easy to resolve. He required a short series of treatments with Active Release Techniques to release the restrictions in his tissues. This was accompanied by a combined series of jaw, neck, shoulder, core, and hip exercises that helped to increase flexibility in restricted structures, increase strength in weakened structures, and retrain his neuromuscular systems.

In Josh's case, his jaw and neck pain was primarily due to kinetic chain compensations caused by other problems in his body. Today, Josh is playing for a semi-professional team with no re-occurrence of these problems.

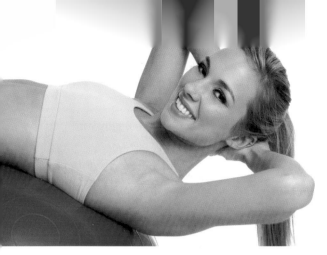

Why Exercise?

Why exercise...a commonly asked question...and one with a multitude of answers. Our bodies evolved to suit an active life, whether the activity was hunting, walking, running, gardening, dancing, farming, chasing children, or playing. Our ancient ancestors did not need exercise programs to keep them fit and healthy; their nomadic or agricultural lifestyle required lots of activity just to stay alive. Even food preparation required a great deal of hard manual labor.

Unfortunately, our modern sedentary lifestyle does not keep our bodies tuned and in good health. To compensate, we must exercise, preferably on a daily basis. That's right...DAILY! Exercise is also critical for recovery from any type of injury. So what are some of the benefits of exercise? Here are just a few!

- Exercise makes you more flexible, giving you a greater range of motion and keeping your body young and supple.

- Exercise strengthens your muscles, making you stronger and more able to perform your daily activities with authority and confidence.

- Exercise keeps you youthful by helping you to lose excess weight by raising your metabolism.

- Exercise gives you a better sense of balance, more stable joints, better posture.

- Exercise helps to curb depression and brings a lot of joy into your life.

- Exercise is essential for tissue repair and recovery from injuries.

- Exercise makes your heart stronger and your circulatory system more efficient! It helps deliver more oxygenated blood to more parts of your body.

- Exercise helps to prevent heart attacks, strokes, cancer, arthritis, and a host of other diseases.

- Exercise helps you to reduce stress, improve immune functions, increase levels of growth hormones, and improve sexual function.

- Exercise releases natural endorphins, the feel good hormones that are released when eating chocolate, or having sex!

- The right combination of exercises can resolve chronic injuries.

If you are serious about your health, then exercise should be an essential component of your daily routine!

Exercise and Tissue Repair

To get a better understanding of why exercise is so essential, let us consider just one of the above benefits – *tissue repair*. The process of tissue repair (after an injury) typically occurs over three distinct phases[1]:

> **Phase One: Reaction or Acute Inflammatory phase** - This 72 hour phase is characterized by swelling and pain. During this phase, use ice to reduce inflammation, and if required, take an over-the-counter anti-inflammatory medication. Avoid using these medications after the first 72 hours since they can have a negative effect on tissue regeneration. Even during this initial stage, it is important to get some motion into the affected area in order to speed the healing process.

> **Phase Two: Regenerative or Repair phase** - During this 48 hour to six-week phase, collagen is formed and laid down to repair the injured area. If the injured person is

---

1.   Acute soft tissue injuries-A review of the Literature, Medicine and Science in Sports and Exercise. Oct. 1986;18(5):489-500. John Kellett

performing the correct exercises, the majority of the collagen will be laid down in the same direction as the tissue being repaired, making the repaired tissue stronger and more capable of performing its function. If the individual is not exercising, the tissue will be laid down in more random patterns, leading to the development of weaker tissue that is easily re-injured.

Phase Three: Remodeling phase - The remodeling phase can last up to 12 months. During this phase the collagen fibers increase in size, diameter and strength. The amount of remodeling that takes place is dependant upon the forces that are applied to the tissue - in other words - the collagen remodels to withstand the stresses that are placed up on it. *Tissue remodeling is dependant on the forces that are applied the tissue. If the injured person is performing appropriate strengthening exercises, the collagen will remodel to withstand the stresses placed upon it.* With exercise, this remodeling will lead to a complete recovery of the injured tissue, along with a decreased chance of re-injury. Without appropriate strength training, the possibility of re-injury is very high.

It is very important to exercise throughout all stages of tissue repair. Lack of exercise results in decreased oxygen levels in soft tissues, increased scar tissue formation, increased muscle atrophy, and can prevent full recovery from the injury.

Benefits of Body Awareness Exercises

To really heal your body or improve its performance, it is necessary to build a good understanding and awareness of your body – from where your muscles and joints are, to your posture, body position, and your sense of equilibrium.

By becoming consciously aware of your body, you will improve your ability to guide your body through these exercises and be able to focus your mind and energy upon the areas that you are trying to strengthen and develop.

As you perform each exercise, think about the specific change that you want to achieve, visualize that change occurring, and visualize your body performing at its best. With each exercise, you need to be totally present in both mind and body. Do not let your mind pull you away from your workouts with thoughts of all the things you have to do today. Your complete focus and attention upon the activity that you are performing will give you immediate and powerful results in performance and development. This is a common technique used by many athletes as they endeavour to reach their peak potential.

You will be amazed at just how powerful this sense of awareness is, and how quickly you can achieve your fitness and health goals. This internal focus and awareness is also a great way to release the stresses of your daily life, which in turn helps you to heal faster.

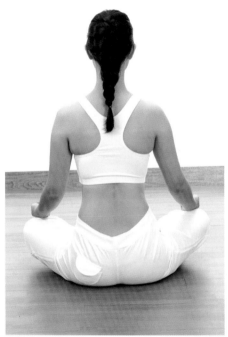

Benefits of Stretching Exercises

Stretching (where you increase the length of your muscles and tendons) is critical for increasing your range of motion and flexibility, improving performance, decreasing the risk of injury, and preventing soreness – not to mention that stretching makes you feel good (just look at the pleasure your pets get when they stretch)!

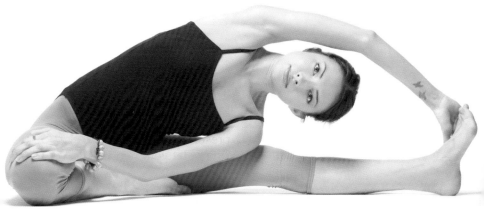

Stretching is particularly important if you have not been exercising on a regular basis, or if you have been training too hard. In such cases, your muscles will tend to contract and shorten due to the sudden strain, and become more prone to injury.

Remodelling tissues with stretches...

During the regenerative or repair phase of an injury, your body creates and lays down collagen to repair the injured area. When the injured person performs the correct stretching exercises, the majority of new tissue will be laid down in the same direction as the tissue that is being repaired - thereby allowing this tissue to properly perform its function (once the healing phase is complete).

Stretching in our exercise program...

Our exercise programs use a combination of static stretches, resistance stretches, and PNF stretches. As you work through the stretches in our book, feel free to customize the routines to work better for you. You may need to change the angle of your stretch to obtain the maximum benefit from the exercise. Try to stretch until you feel a slight pulling sensation (but not pain). *Hold* that position until the stretched muscle relaxes. Increase the stretch each time.

Use your breath to help you stretch and lengthen your tissues. Always *exhale* as you lengthen the tissue, or as you move into the stretch. Slow breathing helps to relax your body, increases blood flow, and facilitates the removal of lactic acid. This is achieved by the rhythmic motion of your lungs (your respiratory pump) as it depresses your diaphragm causing a downward force on your internal organs. This classic Yoga and Tai Chi principle has a very positive effect on your circulatory function.

Bouncing (or ballistic motions) can cause your muscles to suddenly contract when stretched again, causing increased risk of injury. However, there are some stretches that require small bounces, but these are usually used for dynamic warm-ups in athletic or performance training. Do *not* bounce when performing the stretching exercises in this book.

Benefits of Strengthening Exercises

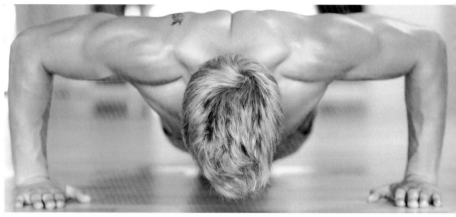

Strength training is a critical component of any exercise program. Unfortunately, strength training is also an area that is often misunderstood and misapplied in many exercise routines. True strength involves neuromuscular control, good body mechanics, correct posture, and excellent core stability. Problems arise if you focus on developing strength without first establishing these preliminary components. Starting strength training too soon can set you up for an injury or result in a decrease in your overall physical performance.

This is why we do not emphasize strength training during the early phases of our exercise routines. Strength training is only introduced after you have mastered the key aspects of our *Beginner Routines* (neuromuscular development, postural changes, and core stability).

On the other hand, once you have established these basics, the benefits of strength training are considerable. Not only will strength training allow your muscles to work harder and longer without injury, it will increase your lean tissue mass, decrease your fat levels, increase your bone density, increase your metabolism, and promote some very positive biochemical changes.

Biochemically, strength training is one of the key factors that will naturally increase your levels of *Human Growth Hormone (HGH)*. This increase is known as the *EIGR Response* or *Exercise Induced Growth Hormone Response.*

As we age, the levels of HGH naturally decrease. This is unfortunate since decreased secretion of growth hormone is (in part) responsible for decreases in lean body mass, increases of adipose-tissue mass (fat), and the thinning of the skin that occur with old age.[1] Obviously, it would be a great thing if we can stop these negative effects from occurring in our body.

The sad truth is that as most people age, they do not focus upon strength training. This is unfortunate since strength training is one of the key tools you can use in turning back your biological clock.

Remodelling tissues with strengthening exercises

Another key reason for strength training has to do with *tissue remodeling.* Every time you injure yourself, your body lays down new tissue to repair itself. The new tissue is initially very fragile, thin, and easily torn or re-injured. Strength or weight training places stress upon these new tissues, causing them to go through a process of remodeling. In this process, the new tissue literally converts from one type of collagen to a different type which is up to 10x thicker and 10x stronger. But, this collagen conversion only occurs when you apply continued stress upon the tissue... as you do in weight and strength–training exercises.

The amazing thing is that this remodeling of your tissues can, with the right stimulus, happen at any age, even for those in their 80's or 90's. Increased age is not an excuse for avoiding strength training exercises. In fact, increasing age often means you need to focus

---

1. Effects of Human Growth Hormone in Men Over 60, New England Journal of Medicine 1990; (323:1-6.)

more on this often neglected area. So, no matter what your age or physical condition, you need to make strength training into an essential part of your exercise routines.

Strengthening in our exercise program...

The strengthening exercises in this book provide you with a path for gradually strengthening your body. Follow this graduated path to increase your strength without over-stressing or injuring your tissues. If you are planning on developing along the path of athletic performance, you may also want to look at our *Release Your Kinetic Chain – Back, Core, and Hips Exercise Book* which is available online at www.releaseyourbody.com.

Benefits of Cardiovascular Exercises

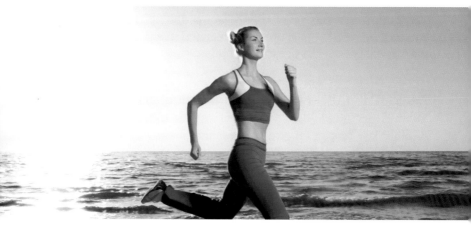

Cardiovascular or aerobic exercises provide huge benefits to your circulatory, respiratory, and immune systems. Aerobic exercises play a key role in speeding healing, increasing performance, preventing degenerative conditions, and even preventing numerous types of cancer.

Weight-bearing exercises such as running and walking strengthen not only your muscles, but also your skeletal system, and help to decrease the risk of osteoporosis and other age–related diseases.

Aerobic or **cardiovascular** exercise is all about increasing your aerobic capacity, improving circulatory function, and increasing energy production. Aerobic exercise does this by increasing the density of capillaries in your muscles and by increasing the level of mitochondrial function in your cells. When you have more capillaries, your cells are able to obtain more nutrients for repair and work, and are able to get rid of waste by-products much more rapidly.

Your mitochondria are the principal energy producers in your cells. Mitochondria convert nutrients into ATP (adenosine triphosphate), a readily–metabolized form of energy used by all living cells. The more energy you have, the easier it is for your body to heal itself and power all the tasks you must perform each day.

Aerobic exercises also promote the loss of excess fat and increases your metabolic rate. In addition, aerobic exercises increase the sensitivity of your cells to insulin, and help your body to better regulate its sugar levels. This is very important for all of us to keep in mind since over 7% of our population now suffers from diabetes; and with increasing rates of obesity, more people are at risk than ever before.

Anaerobic exercise (exercising with reduced blood oxygen levels) is also very important for performance or athletic training. Just like weight training, anaerobic training also promotes the production of Human Growth Hormone (HGH). Research has shown that short intense bursts of anaerobic activity produces high levels of lactic acid. In a high–lactic acid environment, your body increases production of HGH. This means that when we combine anaerobic activity with weight training, we can substantially increase our HGH levels. Bottom line: we will be stronger, leaner, fitter, and healthier.

You should include at least half an hour to forty-five minutes of walking and running in your *daily* exercise regime. If your schedule is too busy for daily walking, then try to ensure that you walk or run vigorously at least three to four times a week. Ideally, you should do this cardiovascular exercise *before* you perform the strengthening and stretching exercises in this book.

Aerobic Warm-Ups...how they helped resolve my injury!

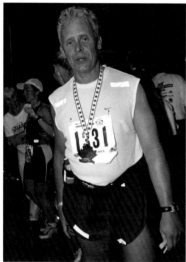

I have had a personal experience that showed me the importance of cardiovascular warm-ups as they relate to recovering from an injury.

I am speaking about an injury for which most people would never perform an aerobic workout. A few years ago I suffered from a severe case of *Bell's Palsy* (weakness of the nerve that enervates and controls the muscles for facial expression) on one-half of the face.

Dr. Abelson, looking a little tired after finishing the Canadian Ironman.

Bell's Palsy left me with the muscles of one-half of my face paralyzed and expressionless. I was told it would take 3 to 6 months before normal nerve function would be restored!

I was unwilling to live with this condition for that long and immediately researched means for reducing this time frame! One of the first things I did after getting Bell's Palsy was to get on my road bike/wind trainer for at least 20 to30 minutes each day. I followed this up with TMJ massage and a variety of jaw, neck, and shoulder exercises.

To everyone's amazement, I recovered fully, with complete neuromuscular control of the muscles in my face within about a month. I am convinced that my daily aerobic exercise is one of the major reasons I got over this condition in about a third of the normal time. The aerobic exercises I did everyday resulted in increased circulatory function and improved mitochondrial activity (energy production)!

So take the time to do your aerobic warm-up before doing these exercise programs...you will be amazed at the difference it makes in your healing, recovery, power, and strength development!

So what is a good warm-up?

A good warm-up should include all the large muscles of your body and include movements that increase your heart rate and breathing. This is a good opportunity to *listen* to your body, and recognize any injury, tight spots, or restrictions that you may have to accommodate during your exercise routine.

- **Go for a brisk 10 to 20 minute walk.** Make sure you move your shoulders and swing your arms. Good upper extremity motion takes the stress off your back and helps you to store and release energy from your core. Don't walk at a slow pace, this will not achieve the desired results and is actually quite hard on your back compared to brisk walking.

- **Jog, or run for 10 to 20 minutes.** If you are not a runner, start with a brisk walk interspersed with a few short jogs. If you are a runner, make sure you maintain a good upright posture with good shoulder movement, and make sure you land on the middle of your feet. No toe or heel running as this deactivates your gluteals and causes a lot of other problems. Treadmills are fine but do not increase your elevation too much.

- **Swim for 20 minutes.** If you are doing the front crawl, make sure you breathe from both sides. I don't want your warm-up to create neuromuscular imbalances because you breathe from just one side of your body.

- **Use an elliptical or ski machine for 10 to 20 minutes.** Both are good for reinforcing a cross-crawling pattern, which helps establish good neuromuscular control, as well as for warming up all the big muscles of your body.

- **Ride a stationary bike for 10 to 20 minutes.** This option is not my first choice due to the lack of motion in the upper extremity. In terms of bike types, I prefer the use of upright bikes much more since you can maintain better posture, especially if you have a history of back pain.

- **Hula-hoop for 5 to 10 minutes.** Most people may not think of this as an aerobic exercise, but it is! The hula-hoop is not only a lot of fun, but it is also a great way to learn how to properly brace your core, a key concept in core stability.

Working within your Aerobic Zone

Your warm-up, like all initial aerobic activity, needs to be performed within your aerobic zone. This is the range within which you want your heart to operate while you are performing your aerobic exercise. Think of your aerobic zone as the base which you must first establish for rehabilitation, and also for moving into the higher levels of performance in your chosen activity.

Calculating your aerobic zone - Use the following formula to calculate your *aerobic zone*:

1. Subtract your age from the number **220**.
    - For example, if I am **40** years old, then **220 - 40 = 180**.
2. Obtain the low end of your aerobic range by multiplying the result of step1 by **0.6**.
    - In our example: **180 * 0.6 = 108**
3. Obtain the high end of your aerobic range by multiplying the result of step1 by **0.7**.
    - In our example: **180 * 0.7 = 126**

This is your *aerobic heart rate zone* within which you need to work to develop your aerobic capacity. It is the zone which will best speed your recovery from an injury. If you work above this zone you run the risk of injury. If you work below this zone, you will not achieve the maximum benefits provided by your aerobic warm-up.

Benefits of Proprioceptive Exercises

Proprioception or balance is something we take for granted – that is, until we lose it! In our youth, we all had fantastic balance and had a natural sense of our position and place in space. We thought nothing of walking across a narrow beam, or jumping from rock to rock. But as we age, we lose that superb sense of balance, and have to work to regain it!

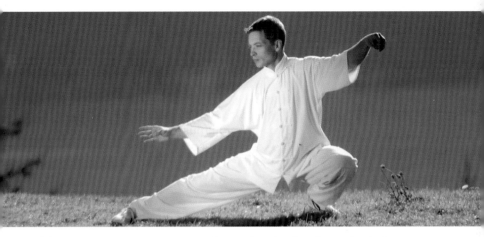

The proprioceptive exercises in our books (such as single leg stances or exercises on a ball) help to increase your stability (from the head, through the neck, shoulders, arms, core, legs, knees, ankles, and feet).

Proprioceptive exercises help you to maintain your balance when you stumble, trip over a rock, or start to fall. Proprioceptive or balance training is a fundamental requirement that should not be ignored in either Rehabilitation Therapy or Sports Performance training. Your ability to balance depends on feedback from your auditory, visual, proprioceptive (sense of body position), and vestibular systems (relating to the sense of equilibrium). All of these systems must be trained to achieve optimal results.

A great way to increase your proprioception is to perform a familiar exercise with your eyes closed. This is a common practice that we use when teaching Tai Chi. Even well-trained athletes are surprised how difficult an easy exercise becomes when their eyes are closed.

Start working on your proprioception early in life, and you may never have to worry about losing your balance and getting hip fractures in your old age. Even better, since proprioceptive exercises are all about learning to recruit more of your nervous system, you will find that your overall sports performance will start to improve as you perform proprioceptive exercises. Remember, the best athletes in the world are defined by their superb neuromuscular control, and this control is what proprioceptive exercises can deliver for you!

What's Special About Our Exercises

The exercises in this book have been selected to help you to develop great neuromuscular control, flexibility, power, and strength in your body. These exercises are very effective in preventing and treating soft tissue injuries if they are performed during the early stages of injury or restriction. These exercises are also key to strengthening the weak links in your kinetic chain. These weak links may have been inhibiting not only your activities of daily living, but also your athletic performance.

Remember, if you have a problem or restriction in any area, then you must first resolve that problem before embarking into Performance training. Otherwise you increase the risk of re-injuring yourself.

- Use the warm-up exercises to relax your body, centre and clear your mind, and prepare your body for the remainder of the exercise routine.

- Use the balance and proprioceptive exercises to develop your neuromuscular control. We cannot over-state the importance of this key factor for both rehabilitation and athletic performance.

- Use the stretching exercises to decrease muscle tension, increase relaxation, increase flexibility, and reduce the risk of muscle, joint, ligament, and tendon injuries.

- Use the resistance exercises to strengthen your bones, muscles, ligaments, tendons and connective tissue.

Through our clinical experience, we have found that the patients who follow our rehabilitative exercise recommendations find that their condition resolves much more quickly. So, don't pick and choose only one exercise. Each routine we recommend combines an optimum collection of exercise types that should be carried out together for the best benefit.

Exercise Accessories and Tools

Although most of our exercises can be performed at home, some of them do require additional accessories or tools. (Most of these exercise accessories/tools can be purchased at www.fitter1.com.) The primary tools that you may need to purchase include:

This equipment	Is used for...
Exercise Handball	Exercise handballs are used to strengthen your fingers, hand, wrist, and arm. The firm grasping action that is required throughout the exercise activates the muscles of the entire upper-extremity kinetic chain. You can obtain different weights and sizes of exercise handballs. Pick one between 3 lb to 5 lb.
Swiss Exercise Ball	Swiss Exercise Balls are those giant balls that you see people bouncing around on. They are also known as Fitness Balls or Balance Balls. Exercising with these Fitness Balls increases your balance, core strength, and proprioception. Ensure that the exercise ball is burst-resistant and the correct size for your height. For example, if you are under 5′8″, then use a 55 cm exercise ball. If you are taller than 5′8″, use a 65 cm exercise ball.
Medicine Balls	Weighted medicine balls can help you to improve your hand-eye coordination, and increase strength, coordination, dynamic flexibility, reaction time, and explosive strength. They range in weight from 5 to 50 lb, and are used in our exercise routines for stretching, abdominal exercises, and strengthening.
Exercise Tubing	The stretchy exercise tubing is used for resistance therapy and strength conditioning. The tubing allows you to adjust the tension to suit your current level of strength and tolerance. As you become stronger, you can shorten the tubing to increase the tension. Ensure you move slowly and smoothly, without any sudden jerky motions.

This equipment	Is used for...
Free Weights	We recommend using free weights (instead of machines) for strengthening exercises. Machines slow your progress and cause injuries by creating abnormal neuro-muscular responses. Machines also give a false sense of strength and power development since they compensate for actions that you would normally be unable to complete with free weights. In contrast, free weights force you to use accessory muscles for balance, and recruit more of your nervous system for better neuro-muscular control. As discussed earlier, the amount of power you are able to generate is directly proportional to the efficiency of your nervous in controlling muscular system action. Adding extra weight causes your muscles to work harder, burn more calories, and improve muscle power and strength. Some key points: • Select a weight that causes your muscles to tire after three sets. • Allow a day of rest between each session of free weight exercises. • Move slowly and smoothly without sudden jerky motions.
Foam Rollers	We use foam rollers in our exercise routines to loosen muscles, release tension, and increase flexibility through the process of Myofascial Release. Foam rollers are a great tool to improve the quality of your tissues since they help to break down fibrous adhesions that form in your muscles after repetitive motions, injury, poor posture, or compensations throughout your kinetic chain. By breaking down these adhesions you increase your body's ability to store and release energy. This allows you to perform exactly the same action, but with much less effort. Best of all, foam rollers can be used to release adhesions from your neck, shoulders, arms, back, hip, legs, and even your feet. Most foam roller exercises start at the origin of the muscle, and move down across the body of the muscle. When a point of tension is reached, hold that position for a few minutes, using your body's weight to cause the muscle to fully relax.

When Exercise Isn't Enough!

Are you dealing with a soft tissue or joint injury that is not resolving from just exercises? Sometimes, your body needs a little more help than what exercise can provide.

In most cases, sprains, strains, muscle spasms, and a wide range of other minor soft tissue injuries often resolve after just seven to ten days with the right exercises and a little self-therapy. Don't get discouraged if this does not occur for you. It is not that the exercises are ineffective; it may just be that you have built up adhesions or scar tissues between your soft tissues that need to be released before the exercises can take effect.

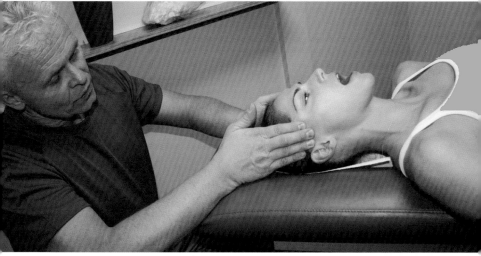

Dr. Abelson releasing TMJ restrictions with Active Release Techniques.

In such cases, it is advisable to seek professional help in releasing these restrictions.

Look for a good Active Release Techniques, Graston Techniques, or Registered Massage Therapy practitioner in your area, or a proficient deep tissue therapist. Keep in mind that numerous Chiropractors, Physiotherapists, Osteopaths, and Occupational Therapists may also be trained in these techniques. So ask questions, and find someone who can help you!

Try the exercises first. If you do not achieve the desired result, then seek professional help. Once the restrictions and adhesed tissues have been released with a technique such as Active Release, exercises will once again become a very effective part of the rehabilitative healing process, and can help to ensure the injury does not return. Check with your practitioner, but most specialists will recommend that you continue your exercise program in conjunction with your treatments.

For more information about possible therapies, see the following sections in this book:

- *Active Release Techniques® (ART) - page 196*
- *Graston Techniques® - page 198*
- *Manipulation - page 200*
- *Massage Therapy - page 202*
- *Physiotherapy / Occupational Therapy - page 204*
- *Acupuncture and Traditional Chinese Medicine - page 206*

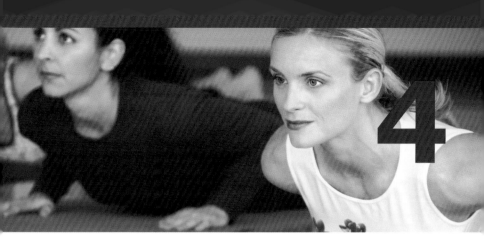

What's Special About These Exercises

Physical training is often poorly executed and misunderstood. All too often people become injured when they are asked to execute extremely challenging training programs without correct preparation of their body. Equally often, I see many athletes trying to work though the pain of their injury only to create a chronic, longer-lasting problem. This situation is usually the direct result of poorly-designed exercise programs.

This may sound strange, but many exercise programs contain components that continue to keep you in your current state of pain, which often cause chronic injuries, and all too often *decrease* your performance.

Good training programs should provide multi-step routines that involve both your **neuromuscular** and **cardiovascular** systems — which together develop your power, balance, flexibility, and strength.

The correct program for you involves much more than just a series of sets, repetitions, and tempo with a few rest days thrown in for good measure. Training is a dynamic program that has to change with the responses of *your* unique body, and that meets *your* specific needs.

Your body is unique and individual - given that each one of us is a unique individual, with specific needs, and unique bodies, you will find that not everyone recovers from an injury at the same rate or within the same time period. Nor will everyone be able to achieve identical levels of athletic performance with the same training program…otherwise we could all be champion athletes.

The key point is, that with our exercise protocols, you can achieve great results if you *closely monitor your body's responses*, and then *fine-tune* the exercise routines accordingly.

Listen to your body - if it tells you to rest, then rest. If your body says you have not yet recovered from your injury, then give it the time it needs. Don't just jump to the next level of training if your body says "*Not Just Yet!*" On the other hand, if your body is sending you the message that it can handle the new demands, then go for it. Just remember that your body may change its mind, so listen to the feedback it is giving you!

Keep your kinetic relationships in mind - remember, the focus of these books is to develop and strengthen not just your individual muscles, but also the inter-relationships between your various soft tissue structures.

For maximum effectiveness, you need to develop an awareness of these kinetic relationships as you perform these exercises. Your conscious awareness of the structural inter-relationships (as you exercise) will have a huge influence upon the effectiveness of these routines.

Take the time to focus and build that body-mind awareness…and thereby improve your neuromuscular control. Remember… *Neuromuscular Control* is the key factor that determines success or failure in your exercise routines.

Progressing Through Our Program

All our *Release Your Kinetic Chain* exercise programs provide a graduated method for rehabilitating and improving your soft tissues (muscles, nerves, tendons, etc). Typically, you will work through the following three or four levels:

- Beginner Routine for 3 to 4 weeks.
- Intermediate Routine for 4 to 6 weeks.
- Advanced Routine for 6 to 8 weeks.
- Performance Development Routines for 4 to 6 weeks or as long as needed.

Before starting with our exercise routines, it is important for you to take the time to determine your current status or stage of training. The answers to the following questions will help you to determine your current level of training and determine which routines are appropriate for you to use. Ask yourself:

- When did you last exercise on a regular basis?
- Is this your first time using exercise routines?
- How long have you been doing your current routine?
- Are you trying to rehabilitate an injury?
- Are you preparing for a sports season or athletic event?

Review your answers against the following categories to determine where you should start in our routines. See:

- *Use the Beginner Routines in this book if: - page 54.*
- *Use the Intermediate Routines in this book if: - page 55.*
- *Use the Advanced Routines in this book if: - page 56.*
- *Use the Performance Routines in this book if: - page 57.*

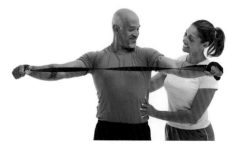

Use the Beginner Routines in this book if:

- ❑ You are recovering from injuries.
- ❑ You have never worked out before.
- ❑ You have limited knowledge about how to get fit.
- ❑ You have taken a long break from exercising and would like to start again.

If you fit this description, then start with our **Beginner Routines**, which emphasize the introduction of:

- ❑ Neuromuscular control.
- ❑ Body awareness.
- ❑ Flexibility.
- ❑ Proprioception.
- ❑ Coordination.

Inactive people often lack the coordination and ability to perform complex motor tasks, largely due to lack of use of their nervous and muscular systems. The *Beginner Routines* emphasize the process of **neuromuscular grooving** where the act of repeatedly performing a specific motion helps your body to learn how to execute that motion well and without conscious attention to that action. These *Beginner Routines* help you to recruit more of your nervous system as you perform each task.

The *Beginner Routines* lay the foundation for coordinating the inter-relationships between your nervous, muscular, and skeletal systems with the goal of helping you to effectively perform any required action.

Use the Intermediate Routines in this book if:

- ❏ You have been exercising three to five times a week.

- ❏ You have achieved a baseline level of endurance.

- ❏ You can easily perform the *Beginner Routines* in this book without pain or effort and feel that you are now ready to progress to the *Intermediate Routines.*

- ❏ Your previous soft tissue or joint injuries have fully resolved.

If you fit this description, then you are ready to use the Intermediate level of our exercise routines to further develop:

- ❏ Neuromuscular control.

- ❏ Coordination.

- ❏ Flexibility.

- ❏ Balance and Proprioception.

- ❏ Endurance.

The recruitment and optimization of your motor systems remains a fundamental component of these routines. This is also when you begin to increase, add, and vary various elements such as weights, sets, repetitions, and levels of difficulty into your routines.

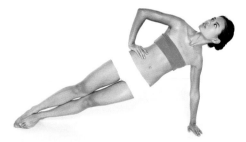

Use the Advanced Routines in this book if:

- ❏ You already participate in physical activity on a regular basis (4 to 6 days per week).
- ❏ You are ready to challenge yourself at a higher level.
- ❏ You are ready to increase the level of performance for a specific sport or activity.
- ❏ You are injury-free.
- ❏ You have already progressed through the *Intermediate Routines* in this book without pain or effort.

These advanced routines incorporate the following elements:

- ❏ Higher levels of neuromuscular control.
- ❏ Increased power generation through the core.
- ❏ Increased strength development.
- ❏ Improved stability and balance.

We incorporate core stabilization exercises at all levels of exercise, with increasing emphasis on this aspect as you advance through each level. For further advanced core exercises, refer to our *Release Your Kinetic Chain – Back, Core and Hip Exercise* book, which focuses on developing all aspects of core stability and performance care.

Remember, for maximum benefits and to prevent injury, you must first be able to comfortably perform the exercises in the *Intermediate Routines* before progressing to the *Advanced Routines*.

Use the Performance Routines in this book if:

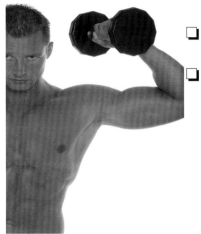

❑ You want to improve your level of athletic performance.

❑ You have reached a plateau in your sport of choice and you want to surpass that plateau.

The majority of the strengthening and stretching exercises at the Performance level are dynamic, oriented towards increasing athletic performance, and require advanced training of your neuromuscular system to allow for smooth, economical performance of basic motions.

Note: This book does *not* focus upon exercises relating to a single or specific sporting activity. Instead, we address universal kinetic chain elements that apply to a broad spectrum of athletic activities. For more focused exercises, refer to our upcoming books – **Release Your Stride** (for runners and walkers) and **Release Your Swing** (for golfers).

How are our routines organized?

Each exercise routine in our book is set up in the following order:

■ Myofascial release (warm-up).
■ Neuromuscular training.
■ Strengthening exercises.
■ Core stabilization exercises.
■ Dynamic and static flexibility exercises.

This order stresses, works, and fatigues the biggest muscles first, and then focuses on working the smaller muscles.

Understanding Repetitions and Sets

Almost all our exercise routines require you to perform a number of repetitions and sets of that exercise. So what are sets and reps?

Repetitions (R) - "Reps" or repetitions are the number of times you repeat a particular action. For instance, when you perform a bicep curl 10 times in a row, then you have essentially performed 10 repetitions of that exercise, also shown as 10R.

Sets (S) - These ten repetitions make up one "set". After each set you should briefly rest (20 to 30 seconds) before starting the next set of repetitions. In our books we will always tell you how many repetitions and sets you should do for each exercise. This information appears on the side of each exercise page as follows:

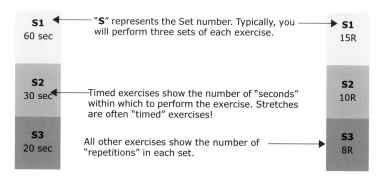

Timed Exercises

Regular Exercises

| S1 60 sec | "S" represents the Set number. Typically, you will perform three sets of each exercise. | S1 15R |

Timed exercises show the number of "seconds" within which to perform the exercise. Stretches are often "timed" exercises!

| S2 30 sec | | S2 10R |

All other exercises show the number of "repetitions" in each set.

| S3 20 sec | | S3 8R |

The above graphic appears on the outside edge of each exercise page, and indicates how many **repetitions** you should perform for each **set**. The **S** indicates the number of **sets** and the **R** indicates the number of **repetitions**. If the exercise is timed, there will be a time period stated within the box, as indicated in the example on the left.

Typically, you start by performing one set of an exercise, and increase the number of sets as you progress. Keep the following points in mind as you perform each exercise:

- *How long should I rest between sets? ....see page 59.*
- *Applying the Inverted Pyramid Structure to your sets ....see page 59.*
- *Setting your Exercise Tempo ....see page 60.*

How long should I rest between sets?

We are often asked how long the rest period should be between each set of exercises. Use the following guide to determine your rest period between sets:

Determining Your Rest Period

Training Level	Rest Period
Beginner Routines	1/2 to 1 minute
Intermediate Routines	1 to 2 minutes
Advanced Routines	2 minutes

Applying the Inverted Pyramid Structure to your sets

With the inverted pyramid structure, select a weight that allows you to comfortably perform the total number of repetitions in the first set. For example, if the first set of an exercise requires you to perform 12 repetitions, then you should select a weight that lets you do this comfortably. For example an inverted pyramid training for a bicep curl may look like the following:

S1 – 12 R

■ Begin by doing 12 repetitions of a bicep curl in the first set.

S2 – 10 R

■ Follow with 10 repetitions in the second set.

S3 – 8 R

■ End with 8 repetitions in the third set.

The Beginner Routines are more concerned with developing your ability to actually perform an action (*motor grooving*) than with the amount of weight you are lifting. Once you progress to the Intermediate/Advanced routines, weight and tension become a more important factor. At this level, you should aim to increase your weight or tension (tubing exercises) by about 10% each week.

Your body tends to adapt and plateau quickly if you perform the same number of exercises, at the same weight/tension every week.

When this occurs, you will not increase in power or strength. Due to this, it is essential to increase the weight/resistance of an exercise on a weekly basis.

By applying the inverted pyramid structure (where the number of repetitions decrease with each subsequent set) you also decrease the chances of injury. The intent of our exercise routines is to increase your power and strength by increasing the load placed on your muscles, not to bring your muscle tissue to the point of failure!

Setting your Exercise Tempo

Setting a good tempo for your exercise routines is very important. People have a natural tendency to approach unfamiliar activities with the "*just wing it*" mind set.

Often, with physical activity, people use momentum to quickly power their body through the action. This is not a good idea. Moving quickly or jerkily through an exercise will cause you to fail in achieving the results you desire, since excessive momentum can strain or tear your muscles, tendons, and ligaments and increases the likelihood of further injury. We often tell our clients, "*Slow and steady wins the race!*" This is especially true with resistance exercises.

If you are performing an exercise routine for the first time:

- Pace yourself.
- Count slowly in your head as you perform the action.

As a general rule, when you are shortening the muscle, you should perform that action slightly faster, but take a longer period as you lengthen the muscle. We typically set our tempo at a ratio of 2:4, with two counts for contraction, and four counts for lengthening.

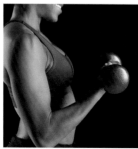

For instance, if you were performing the *Bicep Curl*, you would contract the muscle for a count of two, and then lengthen your arm for a count of four.

You will find that by training with a controlled tempo, you will recruit more muscles during the exercise, and that each repetition provides more effective results.

Frequently Asked Questions (FAQs)

Our patients often ask us many questions when they start our exercise routines. The following are some of the most common questions:

- ❑ *When should I exercise? - page 61*
- ❑ *Can I eat or drink before exercising? - page 62*
- ❑ *What is a Concentric vs. Eccentric Contraction? - page 63*
- ❑ *How often should I exercise? - page 64*
- ❑ *How long do I have to stay at each level of exercise? - page 63*

When should I exercise? - It is best to avoid performing strenuous exercises early in the morning since the likelihood of injury increases after a long period of inactivity (sleep) when your muscles are still stiff and cold. If you want to exercise in the morning, then start with a good warm-up, such as a brisk walk for 10 to 20 minutes before progressing to your routines.

According to several studies, the ideal time to workout is during the late afternoon when your body is at its peak strength.[1]

A workout later in the day is advantageous for the following reasons:

- ■ Decreased likelihood of injury.
- ■ Increased hormones.
- ■ Increased nutrient levels.
- ■ Increased blood flow.
- ■ Decreased metabolism and energy levels.

One of the exercises we do recommend for the early morning is the **Cat Stretch** (page 138) which should be performed first thing in the morning, just after getting out of bed. The flexion and extension motion of the spine that occurs during this exercise creates a pumping action which acts to displace fluid collecting in the discs of your vertebrae.[2] This has a positive effect in reducing even chronic back pain.

1. Wendy Bumgardner. What's the Best Time of Day to Exercise? March 5, 2008. http://walking.about.com/od/fitness/a/besttimeex.htm
2. Stuart M. McGill, Enhancing Low Back Health through stabilization exercise. University of Waterloo. http://www.ahs.uwaterloo.ca/~mcgill/fitnessleadersguide.pdf

Can I eat or drink before exercising? - Just like your car needs fuel to drive, your body needs a good supply of nutrients to perform at its best! You should eat a light, healthy snack approximately two hours before physical activity (it takes approximately one to two hours to digest a snack). Then eat a healthy meal within one hour after exercising, or have a shake comprised of an isolate whey protein combined with L-Glutamine.

It is important to stay well hydrated while exercising. Take small sips of water frequently during activity. Strenuous activity leads to dehydration and depletion of essential electrolytes and minerals.

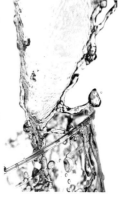

Even a few percentage-points drop in your fluid levels can lead to substantial decreases in performance caused by decreases in oxygen delivery and a build-up of lactic acid by-products. This can lead to symptoms such as dizziness, and nausea.

If you are active and dehydrated, you could get heat stroke, especially if you are outdoors and in a warmer climate. After exercising, drink plenty of water to move toxins away from your active muscle tissue.

In general terms, you should drink approximately 8 to 10 glasses of water each day. Actual amount consumed should increase when you are in high-temperature environments or are performing intense or demanding exercise routines.

Good quality electrolyte-replacement drinks can also aid in rapid recovery. Avoid high-fructose drinks since they have a tendency to spike your sugar levels. Electrolyte–replacement drinks such as Endurox-R4 and Cytomax provide a good balance of electrolytes, carbohydrates, and protein, allowing for increased performance and faster recovery.

For more information about diet and nutrition please refer to the *Kinetic Health Nutritional Program*, available on our websites.

What is a Concentric vs. Eccentric Contraction? - The shortening and lengthening of a muscle involve two different types of contractions – concentric and eccentric.

During a typical strengthening exercise, the first part of the action involves a **concentric contraction**, where **both sides of the muscle come together to shorten the tissue.** This is common for lifting actions, such as the bicep curl.

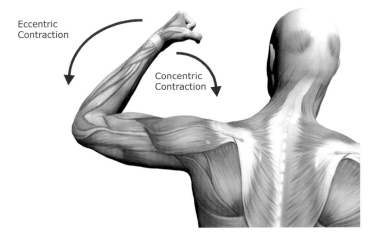

Eccentric
Contraction

Concentric
Contraction

An **eccentric contraction** occurs when the muscle tissue moves the ends of the muscle **away** from each other, lengthening the muscle. This motion is often responsible for returning the muscle to its starting position.

In strength training, eccentric contractions provide the most effective means for gaining strength and size in the muscle. This is why we recommend, in any individual exercise, that you take more time to perform eccentric contractions, and less time to perform concentric contractions.

How long do I have to stay at each level of exercise? - When you repeat the same exercise routine continually, you will find that your body adapts and that the benefits of that routine diminish. This is known as a *plateau effect*, where your body has adapted to the demands you place and is no longer improving or increasing in strength, even though you continue to exercise.

For example, many of our patients perform physically demanding jobs and inform us that their work is their main form of physical exercise. In such cases, it is important for our patient to recognize that their body has already adapted to the physical demands of the job, and that their work cannot be considered a form of physical exercise.

To avoid this "plateau effect" and to decrease boredom, you should change your exercise routines regularly. This is the main reason we have structured our routines to include increasing levels of difficulty. Typically we recommend that you spend:

- ❏ 3 to 4 weeks in the *Beginner Routines.*
- ❏ 4 to 6 weeks in the *Intermediate Routines.*
- ❏ 6 to 8 weeks in the *Advanced Routines.*
- ❏ 4 to 6 weeks in the *Performance Care Routines.*

Once you reach the Performance Care level, you may want to retain the services of a Personal Trainer or Coach to help you develop additional exercise routines that help you to achieve your fitness goals.

How often should I exercise? - This is a commonly asked question at our clinic. The frequency of exercise often depends on the type of activity. As a general rule of thumb, you should:

- Perform cardiovascular activity every day for at least 20 to 30 minutes. And yes, Saturday and Sunday are also included in the "daily" prescription. Cardiovascular activity should take place *before* starting any other exercise routine.

- Perform dynamic range of motion exercises to get your mind and body working together, before beginning any other component of your exercise routine. This activates your neuromuscular system.

- Perform weight-bearing exercises on alternate days. Give yourself a day of rest in-between to give your body a chance to rest, repair, and recover from the previous day's workout.

- Perform flexibility and stretching exercises daily. Ideally a total body stretch of 10 to15 minutes should occur at the end of your workout.

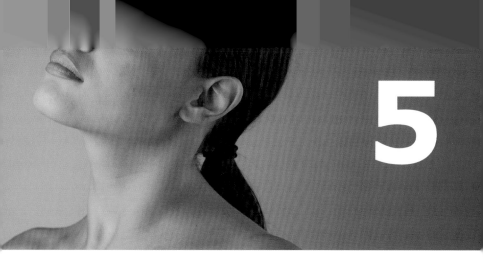

5

What's your problem... Jaw and TMJ?

You use it thousands of times a day, and don't even think about it! Your jaw is involved in every conversation you have, every meal you eat, and every bite you take. When the muscles of your jaw, neck, or shoulders become tight, restricted, or injured, it becomes difficult or impossible to perform vital daily tasks such as chewing food and speaking.

Ask yourself:

■ Does your jaw feel stiff or locked?

■ Do you have difficulty chewing, yawning, or talking?

■ Do you have difficulty opening your mouth?

■ Do you notice a clicking, grinding, or popping sound when you open your mouth?

■ Do you suffer from frequent earaches (just in front or below the ear) that are NOT caused by an infection?

■ Do you have frequent headaches or neck aches?

■ Is your jaw stiff and sore in the morning when you wake up?

■ Have you ever injured your jaw or neck?

If you answered YES to one or more of the above questions, you may be suffering from a soft tissue injury to the muscles and tissues of your jaw and neck. Common jaw problems that cause pain include:

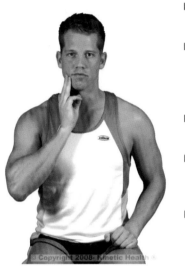

- Temporomandibular Joint Dysfunctions (TMD or TMJ).

- Bruxism, or grinding of your teeth, which can also cause problems in the alignment of your teeth.

- Dental treatments that result in tight, inflamed jaw muscles.

- Jaw pain due to trauma, accidents, or other minor injuries.

- Myofascial pain due to restrictions in the muscles of the jaw, neck, and shoulder.

During the early stages of these jaw injuries, mobilization exercises can help to relieve many of these symptoms and restore function to your jaw. After all, it is always nice to be able to chew and eat comfortably!

TMJ or TMD...what is it?

The Temporomandibular Joint (TMJ) lies just in front of the ears, where the lower jaw hinges. If this joint and its accompanying soft tissues are restricted or unbalanced, it can cause conditions such as headaches, earaches, facial pain, vision problems, eye pain, teeth problems, balance issues, tinnitus, throat and neck pain, dizziness, and a host of other symptoms.

TMJ (Temporomandibular Joint Syndrome) and TMD (Temporomandibular Joint Disorder) are two of the most common causes of facial pain. (The most common cause of facial pain is actually a toothache!) Jaw pain, typically related to the TMJ, is often caused by stress (mental or physical).There are two distinct types of TMJ dysfunctions, both of which can be present at the same time:

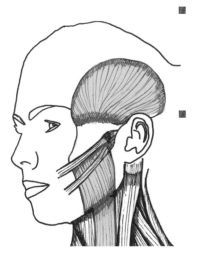

■ **Muscle-related TMJ**: This type of TMJ often results from myofascial pain and dysfunction (MPD). The exercises you will find in this book can help you to find relief from this type of TMJ.

■ **Articular or Joint-related TMJ**: This type of TMJ is due to articular or joint disease and is best treated by your dentist. Articular TMJ often has a secondary muscular component that needs to be addressed in order to obtain full resolution of the problem.

Obviously, if you suffer from a combination of both these types of TMJ, your treatment and resolution process will be more complex and challenging.

Since this is basically an exercise book, we will focus on using exercises to relieve and release specific muscles and connective tissues that are involved in Muscle-related TMJ. You can probably obtain considerable relief and substantial results by dealing with this soft tissue component (an often neglected perspective).

When to Seek Medical Care for your Jaw

The Temporomandibular Joint (TMJ) is a complex and powerful joint. Usually, TMD is not an indication of something serious happening in your body. In most cases all that is required are simple treatments involving self-care practices that focus upon eliminating muscle spasms, and restoring correct coordination and muscle balance.

For more severe cases of TMD, you should consult your dentist as well as a soft tissue practitioner who is trained in treating disorders of the TMJ. We cannot over-emphasize the importance of obtaining a correct diagnosis. For those of you who suffer from chronic TMJ, we have found that a *managed team approach* which integrates the skills of a soft tissue practitioner, a dentist or orthodontist, along with appropriate corrective exercises provides the best benefits.

If your TMJ problem originates from soft-tissue or myofascial restrictions, then you may find exercise, in combination with soft tissue treatments to be the most beneficial method of treatment. This type of TMJ is actually the most common type, and in most cases does *not* show any destructive changes to the TMJ when x-rayed. Soft tissue-related TMD is typically caused by stress, grinding of your teeth (bruxism), or chronic clenching of your jaws.

Under certain circumstances, you should seek medical care for your jaw pain. This is especially true if your TMD is joint-related, since it is important to rule out problems such as systemic arthritic conditions, degenerative joint disorders (DJDs), infections, and tumours.

Other red flags for which you should see your dentist or seek medical help include:

- Blunt force trauma to your jaw or head which could cause cerebral bleeding.

- Ongoing jaw pain accompanied by stiffness, neck pain, and fever, which could be indications of meningitis.

- Severely restricted jaw movements where you are unable to open or close your mouth, and which affects your ability to ingest food.

Note: These severe conditions are very rare compared to the muscle-related varieties of TMD.

Exercises and Recommendations for the Jaw

If your TMJ is related to poor posture, a recent trauma (such as a motor vehicle accident), or is a relatively recent occurrence, then the exercises in this book should help you to resolve your condition quite rapidly. However, do keep in mind that chronic TMJ (that has lasted for many years) will take longer to resolve. This does not mean you cannot achieve very good results. It only means that you will have to commit to performing these exercises for a longer period of time.

Try some of the following exercises to relieve tension in your jaw and neck, and to restore your ability to chew, talk, yawn, and laugh! Yes...you may laugh when you try some of these...and you may feel a little ridiculous doing them, but they do work! So give it a go...and laugh a little while doing them! See the following categories of exercises for more details:

 Warm-up for Your Jaw ....see page 71.

❏ *Beginner's Jaw and TMJ Workout ....see page 72.*

❏ *Intermediate Jaw and TMJ Workout ....see page 73.*

❏ *Advanced Jaw and TMJ Workout ....see page 74.*

In addition to these exercises, consider doing the following:

■ **Apply cold packs**: A cold pack or ice can help to reduce pain, inflammation, or swelling. Apply a cold pack to the affected area of your jaw for about 10 to 15 minutes, two to three times a day. This is especially important immediately after physical trauma.

■ **Get a dental appliance**: Speak to your dentist to determine if a night guard or intra-oral splint can help.

■ **Modify your diet**: Avoid eating hard crunchy foods, or large pieces of food. Until you resolve your jaw problem, try eating soft foods that are cut into small pieces...especially during an acute attack of pain.

■ **Modify your lifestyle**: Avoid chewing gum, biting your nails, or any other activity that further stresses your TMJ.

■ **Apply hot compresses**: Apply a hot pack (or a cloth soaked in warm water) to the area where you feel the most pain or tenderness. Apply the hot pack for about 10 to15 minutes, two to three times a day. **Note**: Do not use hot compresses if there are any indications of inflammation, swelling, heat, or redness.

- **Change your jaw position**: Try to keep your jaw in a relaxed position. One of the best positions for your TMJ is with your teeth slightly apart, lips slightly together, and with your tongue touching the roof of your mouth.

- **Change your posture**: Many people suffer from TMJ simply because of an anterior (head jutting forward) posture. If your job or lifestyle requires you to sit for long periods of time, it is critical to practice good posture. Sit so that your back is straight, ears aligned over your shoulders, and your head slightly erect. Keep your jaw in a relaxed position.

- **Avoid stress**: Yes...stress is a major factor in the majority of TMJ cases. Reduce your stress by practising techniques such as yoga, tai chi, breathing exercises, meditation, or simple walks in natural surroundings.

Note: Advanced cases of TMJ (in which there are many restrictions in the soft tissues of the jaw and neck) may not be fully resolved with just these recommendations and exercises.
In such cases, look for a good soft tissue practitioner (such as an Active Release Techniques practitioner) to help you remove those restrictions. THEN...follow up by doing these exercises on a regular basis to keep the condition from re-occurring!

Watch our YouTube video about TMJ Exercises to learn more about taking care of your TMJ injuries.

1. Start your internet browser application.
2. Navigate to the site *www.youtube.com/kinetichealthonline.*
3. Beside our list of videos, locate the **Search** button and field.
4. Enter the text "**TMJ Exercises**" and click **Search**.
   YouTube will return the name of the video "**TMJ Exercises – Kinetic Health**".
5. Double-click on the video image to start viewing the TMJ video.

We are constantly adding new videos about a wide range of health conditions and about techniques for improving sports and athletic performance. You can also subscribe to our YouTube channel for FREE, so you can stay informed and up-to-date about all our new videos.

Warm-up for Your Jaw

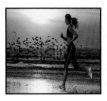

It may sound a little strange, but before beginning any exercise program for your jaw muscles, you should first perform a general, 10-to-15 minutes aerobic warm-up for your entire body. Your goal is to increase your heart rate, get your blood pumping, and prime and ready your body for the next step.

Review —> So what is a good warm-up?, page 43

See *Benefits of Cardiovascular Exercises - page 40* for more details and a better understanding of these benefits! Then do your aerobic warm-up. Follow this up with the relaxation exercises for your jaw!

Massaging the muscles around your jaw can have great benefits. Massage increases circulatory function, delivers more oxygen to your cells, moves nutrients to muscles, displaces by-products of inflammation, and helps to reduce overall pain. Perform the following warm-up massages before starting any jaw exercise routine.

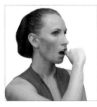

Pterygoid Massage, page 102

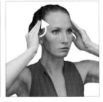

Temporal Massage, page 103

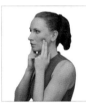

Masseter Massage, page 104

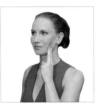

Activate Masseter Trigger Points, page 105

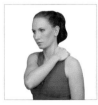

Massage Your Neck and Shoulders, page 119

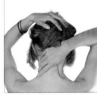

Massage the Back of Your Neck, page 120

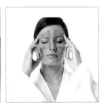

Release Your Sinuses, page 120

Beginner's Jaw and TMJ Workout

Before beginning this Beginners workout, take a few minutes to warm up your body (*So what is a good warm-up? - page 43*) and relax your jaw with the routines and massages shown in *Warm-up for Your Jaw - page 71*.

The exercises in the *Beginner's Jaw and TMJ Workout* should always be performed in a completely pain-free state (as should any rehabilitation protocol). In this routine, you will first work on your neck and shoulders to release restrictions and establish good motor patterns in areas which may affect jaw function. You then move on to some very simple jaw exercises, performed within a **pain-free range**, to help establish positional stability and groove motor-neural patterns.

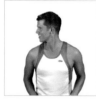

Setting and Activating the Scapulae, page 142

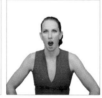

Shoulder Rolls, page 155

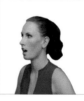

See your Shoes, Watch the Stars, page 125

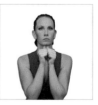

Ears to your Shoulder, page 124

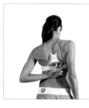

Shoulder Check, page 123

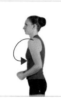

TMJ Opening and Closing, page 116

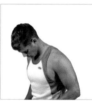

Clicking Your Tongue, page 113

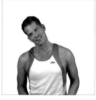

Isometric Jaw Resistance, page 114

Intermediate Jaw and TMJ Workout

Take a few minutes to relax the muscles of your jaw with the routines and massages shown in *Warm-up for Your Jaw - page 71*, and follow this with a short aerobic warm up. Before progressing to this workout you must be able to comfortably perform the exercises in *Beginner's Jaw and TMJ Workout - page 72*, for at least 1 to 2 weeks. Perform the following exercise routines within a **pain-free** zone of safety.

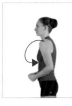

Shoulder Rolls, page 155

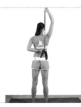

Triceps and Shoulder Stretch, page 147

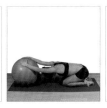

Stretch Your Upper Back, page 128

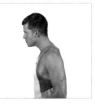

Make Like a Rooster, page 126

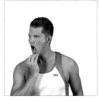

Assisted Opening of the Mouth, page 108

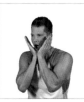

Resisted Opening of the Mouth, page 109

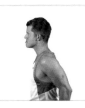

Protracting and Retracting the Jaw, page 110

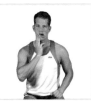

Lateral Mobilization of the Jaw, page 111

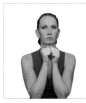

Isometric Jaw Resistance, page 114

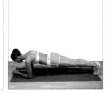

Beginner's Front Bridge, page 159

Advanced Jaw and TMJ Workout

Before progressing to this **advanced** workout, it is essential that you are able to comfortably perform the exercises in *Intermediate Jaw and TMJ Workout - page 73*, for at least 1 to 2 weeks.

Before beginning this advanced workout, take a few minutes to warm up your body and then relax the muscles of your jaw with the routines and massages shown in *Warm-up for Your Jaw - page 71*. Again, all the following exercise routines must be performed in a **pain-free** zone.

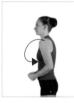
Shoulder Rolls, page 155

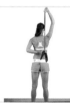
Triceps and Shoulder Stretch, page 147

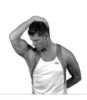
PNF – Stretch your Levator Scapulae, page 136

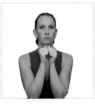
Isometric Jaw Resistance, page 114

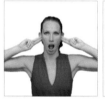
Functional Opening of the Jaw, page 107

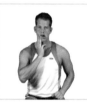
Lateral Mobilization of the Jaw, page 111

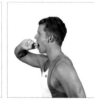
Fist in Mouth... Stretching the TMJ, page 112

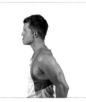
Protracting and Retracting the Jaw, page 110

Strengthen Your Neck with a Swiss Ball, page 137

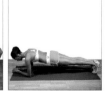
Beginner's Front Bridge, page 159

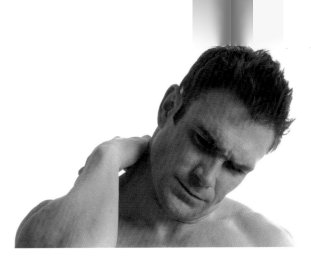
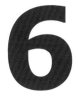

What's your problem...Neck?

Did you know that the human head weighs between 10 to 11 lbs? Well, your neck certainly knows! Not only does your neck carry the weight of your head, it also lets your head turn from side to side and up and down to view the world, and protects those vital nerves and blood vessels that travel from your brain to the rest of your body! However, your neck is less protected than other parts of your spine, and is therefore more vulnerable to injury, and to disorders that restrict motion.

Disorders to the neck, be it a repetitive strain injury (from working on a computer), strained muscles from a whiplash accident, or stress from holding the head in an awkward position (as in a dental office), can result in pain and dysfunction.

Ask yourself:

■ Have you ever suffered from a whiplash accident?

■ Did a sudden motion cause sprain/strain of the tissues in your neck?

■ Do you suffer from frequent tension headaches?

■ Do you have limited range of motion in your neck and shoulders?

■ Do you suffer from chronic stiffness in your neck and shoulders?

■ Does your neck pain affect your activities at home, work, or even sleep?

Neck pain is one of the most common chronic conditions that we treat at our clinic. The good news is that most types of neck pain respond well to the right exercises! The key is to apply the right exercises, at the right time, and with a sound understanding of your neck's kinetic chain relationships.

When to Seek Medical Care for your Neck

Most types of soft tissue injuries to the neck can be self-treated, with common sense, exercise, and perhaps some soft tissue treatments. But, there are some conditions that require prompt medical attention. If you find that you are suffering from any of the following symptoms, **seek *medical attention immediately*,** and *do not* do the exercises in this book until you have had that condition addressed by a skilled medical practitioner.

- Loss of feeling and coordination in your arms and legs.
- Numbness, tingling and weakness in your limbs which could indicate nerve damage and should be addressed promptly.
- Fever, drowsiness, severe headaches, nausea, or vomiting.
- Blunt-force trauma to your neck or head that could cause cerebral bleeding.
- Ongoing neck or jaw pain accompanied by stiffness and fever, which could be indications of meningitis.

Attention: Be safe...not sorry! If you are experiencing neck pain that is accompanied by numbness in your chest, shoulder, or arm, then please **do not** attempt any of the exercises or techniques in this book. You should contact your physician immediately for a proper evaluation.

Note: If you have had neck pain for a long period of time (for over two weeks), you may want to consult a soft tissue specialist **before** beginning an exercise regime. Long-term stress, poor posture, or micro-trauma to the neck can result in the laying down of adhesive tissues that prevent free movement. When this occurs, exercise alone may not be able to restore function. You will need to find someone (such as an Active Release Techniques or Graston Techniques practitioner) who can break these restrictions. Once these restrictions are gone, the exercises in this book can help you to restore full function to your neck.

Preventative Maintenance for Your Neck

Maintain Good Posture - Correct posture is a fundamental requirement for addressing any type of neck problem and involves more than just the position of your neck and head. Proper positioning of your **whole** body is essential, since poor posture in your lower extremities will directly affect the muscles of your neck.

For example, one of the most common **poor posture** stances we see is the "**anterior posture**". In this, the individual exhibits some of the following characteristics:

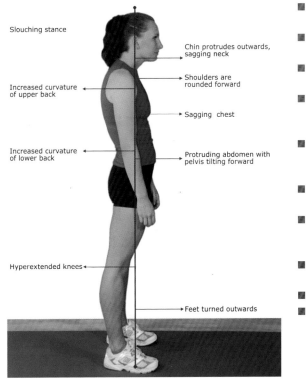

Slouching stance

Increased curvature of upper back

Increased curvature of lower back

Hyperextended knees

Chin protrudes outwards, sagging neck

Shoulders are rounded forward

Sagging chest

Protruding abdomen with pelvis tilting forward

Feet turned outwards

- Chin protruding outwards.
- Forward rounding of the shoulders.
- Drooping front neck muscles.
- Increased curvature of the neck.
- A rounded, sagging or protruding abdomen.
- Head tilting forward and down.
- Increased curvature of the lower spine.
- Pelvis which tilts forward.
- Slouching stance.
- Feet turned outwards.

Having poor posture wastes your energy, causes spinal disc problems, and creates micro-tears in your soft tissues. Poor posture is one of the most common causes of neck, shoulder, and back pain, and can even cause difficulty in breathing.

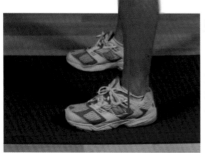

So what is good posture? What should you look for as you try to improve your posture? If you had perfect posture, this is what you would see.

This line would pass through your ear lobe, then directly through the middle of your shoulders, and through the centre of your hip joint, over the side of the knee, and then down to a point about two inches in front of your ankle joint.

How do you achieve this perfect posture? Try this little exercise!

1. Pull your shoulders back and down. *Setting and Activating the Scapulae ....see page 142*

2. Ensure your upper back is relatively flat between the shoulder blades.

3. Your chest curves back, not forward. The forward tips of your shoulder should be one or more inches behind a ruler placed across your upper chest.

4. Your chin is three or more inches above the sternal notch (the small hollow at the base of your neck).

5. Retract or pull back your head just a little so that your ears are aligned directly over your shoulders. To achieve this position, imagine a string pulling your head up towards the ceiling.

6. Extend your hip slightly so that your back muscles are relaxed, and not rigid.

Do you feel the difference? Now try to maintain this posture as you sit, stand and walk.

Get the right pillow - That's right...your pillow could be the cause of your chronic neck pain! Sleeping with too many pillows, or too high a pillow can place stress on the muscles, ligaments, tendons and facet joints of your neck.

A proper orthopedic pillow will support your head in a neutral position, not too high or low. In this position, your spine is aligned and your muscles are totally relaxed, allowing you to get a good night's sleep.

The right pillow varies from one person to the next. We recommend you try out the pillow for a few nights before deciding which is the right one for you.

Change Positions Frequently - If you find that you are sitting or standing for long periods of time, then make it a point to change your position frequently. When sitting for long periods of time, try to use arm-rests to reduce stress and strain. This will help to release tension in the muscles that support your neck and back.

Avoid Awkward Neck Positions - Try to avoid looking down (such as a poorly positioned computer screen), or looking up for extended periods of time. These positions place a great deal of stress on your neck muscles, and prevent you from maintaining good posture.

Practice Good Computer Ergonomics - If your job requires you to spend long hours in front of a computer, then ensure that your monitor is at eye level, that your posture is erect and comfortable, that your hands are well supported, and that your knees lie slightly below your hips. See our **YouTube** video about **Workstation Ergonomics** for more information.
(http://www.youtube.com/watch?v=KUU6FYxE0YU).

Get Proper Rest - It is important to rest and relax your muscles, but complete inactivity is not advised. Most people require a minimum of 8 hours of sleep each night. Any amount less than 6 hours will prevent your body from healing properly. Lack of rest increases inflammation, increases obesity (by up to 32%), decreases immune function, and slows healing. We have often found that getting enough rest is a key factor in resolving our patients' chronic conditions.

Exercises and Recommendations for the Neck

Try some of the following exercises for relieving tension and restoring mobility to your neck:

❏ *Warm-up for Your Neck ....see page 81.*

❏ *Beginner's Neck Workout ....see page 82.*

❏ *Intermediate Neck Workout ....see page 83.*

❏ *Advanced Neck Workout ....see page 84.*

In addition to these exercises, if you currently have pain or inflammation, you may want to first reduce the inflammation using some of the following techniques:

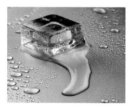

See "Cold Therapy" on page 186.

■ **Apply cold packs:** A cold pack or ice can help reduce pain, swelling, and inflammation from recent injury. Apply a cold pack to the back of your neck for about 10 to15 minutes, two to three times a day.

■ **Apply hot compresses:** Heat treatments should be used for chronic conditions to help relax and loosen tissues, and to stimulate circulation to the area. It can help to increase oxygen levels, transport nutrients in, and transport waste products away.

Apply a hot pack (or a cloth soaked in warm water) to the area where you feel the most pain or tenderness. Apply the hot pack for about 10 to15 minutes, two to three times a day.

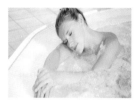

See "Heat Therapy" on page 188.

Note: Do not use hot compresses if there are any indications of inflammation, swelling, heat, or redness.

Warm-up for Your Neck

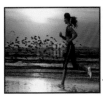

Before starting any of our exercise routines, you need to perform a general cardiovascular warm-up that lasts approximately 10 to15 minutes.

It doesn't matter if this is a brisk walk, a short jog, or riding a bicycle. (See *So what is a good warm-up? - page 43*.) The goal is to raise your body's core temperature enough to increase the elasticity of your muscles, tendons, ligaments, and joint structures. This cardiovascular workout will definitely speed your results and help to prevent any possible injuries that result from over-working cold, stiff muscles.

Review —> So what is a good warm-up?, page 43

Once you have warmed up, you may want to perform one or more of these warm-up massages before starting any neck exercise program to further relax and wake up your neck and shoulder muscles.

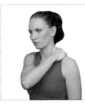

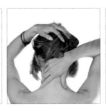

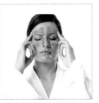

Massage Your Neck and Shoulders, page 119

Massage the Back of Your Neck, page 120

Release Your Sinuses, page 120

Beginner's Neck Workout

Before starting this Beginner's Neck Workout, take a few minutes to warm up your body (*So what is a good warm-up? - page 43*) and relax your neck with the routines and massages shown in *Warm-up for Your Neck - page 81.*

The exercises in the Beginner's Neck Workout should always be performed in a completely pain-free state (as should any rehabilitation protocol). Do these *after* performing the aerobic warm-up and the self-massage. In this routine, we first work on our neck and shoulders to release restrictions and establish good motor patterns in areas that may affect neck function. We then do some very simple isometric neck exercises, within a **pain-free** range, to help establish positional stability and groove motor-neural patterns.

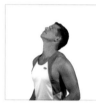

See your Shoes, Watch the Stars, page 125

Ears to your Shoulder, page 124

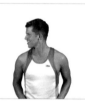

Shoulder Check, page 123

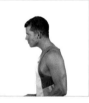

Make Like a Rooster, page 126

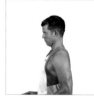

Get that Double Chin, page 127

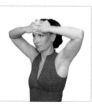

Isometric Neck Resistance, page 130

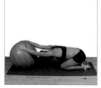

Stretch Your Upper Back, page 128

Foam Roller for Your Neck, page 121

Intermediate Neck Workout

Before progressing to this workout, it is essential that you are able to comfortably perform the exercises in *Beginner's Neck Workout - page 82*, for at least 1 to 2 weeks. Again, all the following exercise routines must be performed in a pain-free zone of safety.

For maximum benefit, before beginning this intermediate workout, take a few minutes to warm up your body (*So what is a good warm-up? - page 43*) and then relax the muscles of your neck with the routines and massages shown in *Warm-up for Your Neck - page 81*.

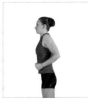
Shoulder Shrugs with Weights, page 154

Shoulder Rolls, page 155

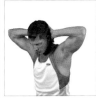
PNF – Flex Your Neck and Head, page 133

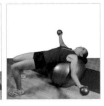
PNF – Extend Your Neck and Head, page 132

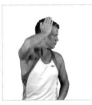
PNF – Cervical Rotation of Your Head, page 135

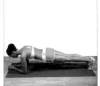
Beginner's Front Bridge, page 159

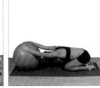
Stretch Your Upper Back, page 128

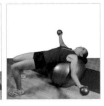
Ball Stretch for the Pectoralis, page 150

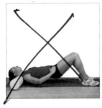
Foam Roller for Your Neck, page 121

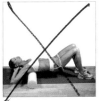
Foam Roller for Your Shoulders, page 149

Advanced Neck Workout

Before progressing to this **advanced** workout, it is essential that you are able to comfortably perform the exercises in *Intermediate Neck Workout - page 83*, for at least 2 to 3 weeks.

Again all the following exercise routines must be performed in a pain-free zone of safety. For maximum benefit, before beginning this intermediate workout, take a few minutes to warm up your body (*So what is a good warm-up? - page 43*) and then relax the muscles of your neck with the routines and massages shown in *Warm-up for Your Neck - page 81*.

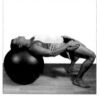
Strengthen Your Neck with a Swiss Ball, page 137

PNF – Flex Your Neck and Head, page 133

PNF – Extend Your Neck and Head, page 132

PNF – Laterally Flex Your Neck and Head, page 134

PNF – Cervical Rotation of Your Head, page 135

PNF – Stretch your Levator Scapulae, page 136

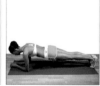
Beginner's Front Bridge, page 159

Beginner's Side Bridge – Knee Bent, page 160

Triceps and Shoulder Stretch, page 147

Lasso with a Handball, page 161

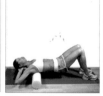
Foam Roller for Your Shoulders, page 149

Foam Roller for Your Neck, page 121

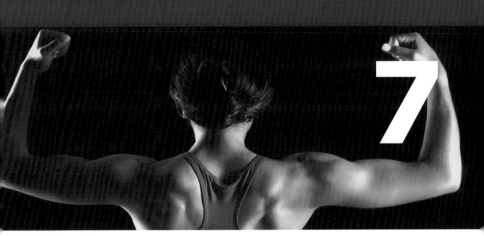

What's your problem...Shoulder?

The inherent instability of the shoulder joint requires us to focus on maintaining a strong, balanced shoulder to prevent injuries and to allow for optimum performance in any sport or other daily activities.

Ask yourself:

- Do you have shoulder pain that has increased gradually over time?

- Have you ever had an injury to your shoulder?

- Do you have pain when you raise or rotate your arms?

- Can you rotate your arm and shoulder through all its normal positions?

- Do you sometimes feel like your shoulder could pop out or slide out of the socket?

- Do you lack the strength in your shoulder to carry out your daily activities?

- Do you have pain at night that prevents you from sleeping on the affected side?

- Do you have numbness or altered sensations in your shoulder?

If you answered YES to one or more of the above questions, you may be suffering from a soft tissue injury to the muscles and tissues of your shoulder. Common shoulder syndromes include:

- Rotator Cuff Injury
- Frozen Shoulder
- Tendonitis
- Thoracic Outlet Syndrome
- Bursitis
- Other Shoulder Impingement Syndromes

These injuries can often be effectively treated with proper exercises, and in chronic cases, with treatments such as:

- *Active Release Techniques® (ART) - page 196*
- *Graston Techniques® - page 198.*
- *Manipulation - page 200.*
- *Massage Therapy - page 202.*
- *Physiotherapy / Occupational Therapy - page 204.*
- *Acupuncture and Traditional Chinese Medicine - page 206.*

By developing good strength in your shoulders, you can:

- Prevent and treat chronic shoulder injuries.
- Address a common source of chronic headaches, neck pain, and jaw pain.
- Improve posture.
- Prevent degenerative arthritic conditions.
- Avoid possible surgical intervention.
- Prevent repetitive strain injuries.
- Improve sport performance in golf, racquet sports, swimming, throwing sports, and many other activities.

When to Seek Medical Care for Your Shoulder

It is sometimes difficult to determine when you need to seek medical attention for a shoulder injury. The majority of shoulder injuries do not always need immediate medical care and can often be healed with time, exercise, and rest. However, we do recommend that you **seek medical attention** if you suffer from one or more of the following symptoms.

Symptoms of Nerve Impingement - These conditions need to be ruled out or addressed by a medical practitioner. Symptoms include:

- Muscle atrophy or substantial decrease in your muscle strength.

- Numbness, tingling, or altered sensation in your shoulder, neck, or down your arm. These signs could indicate nerve impingement, and should be examined and treated by a medical professional or a well-trained soft tissue practitioner.

Symptoms for Cardiovascular Distress - These symptoms need to be ruled out or addressed by a medical practitioner. Symptoms include:

- Shoulder pain that is accompanied by chest pain. This could be an indication of a heart attack if:
  - The chest pain is a squeezing, aching, burning, crushing, or sharp sensation.
  - The chest pain occurs under physical exertion, and decreases when resting.

- Shoulder pain radiating to the left arm or neck.

- Shoulder and chest pain that is linked with shortness of breath.

- Shoulder and chest pain accompanied by symptoms such as breaking out in a cold sweat, nausea, or light-headedness.

Symptoms of physical trauma that should be taken seriously - These conditions need to be ruled out or addressed by a medical practitioner before beginning any exercise program:

- Recent blunt-force trauma.

- Fractures to the bones of the shoulder.

- Dislocation of the shoulder.

- Severe soft tissue damage.

- Bleeding.

Symptoms for shoulder infections are rare - Shoulder infections are rare but need to be considered by your medical practitioner before beginning any exercise program. Symptoms include:

- Redness, swelling, and pain of the tissue with elevated body temperatures above 98.6°F.

- Swelling of the tissues in the shoulder region that cannot be explained by recent physical trauma.

- Recent illness that coincides with the occurrence of the shoulder problem.

Note: If you have had shoulder pain for a long period of time, you may have developed some degree of scar tissue (adhesions) in your shoulder. Long-term stress and trauma to the shoulder can result in the formation of adhesive tissue (scar tissue) that prevent free movement.

When this occurs, exercise by itself may not be able to restore full function. You may need to find someone (such as an Active Release Techniques, Graston Techniques, or Certified Massage practitioner) who can eliminate these adhesions. Once these restrictions are gone, the following exercises can help you to regain motor control, increase muscular endurance and flexibility, and strengthen and restore function to your shoulder.

Don't become discouraged if you have a chronic shoulder problem that does not immediately respond to exercise. Sometimes, even a little therapy can make the exercise work as it should. In our clinic, we commonly treat patients with a history of over 10 years of chronic shoulder problems, and find that they have complete resolution of their problems.

Exercises and Recommendations for the Shoulder

The shoulder routines in this book address all the key aspects of proprioception, motor control, flexibility, and strengthening. It is very important that you carefully follow all the instructions provided with each exercise. These exercises give excellent results when they are performed correctly. But when performed incorrectly, even good exercises can cause problems.

The following pages depict some of the specific exercises that we recommend at our clinic for the rehabilitation of shoulder injuries.

- *Warm-up for Your Shoulder ....see page 90.*
- *Beginner's Shoulder Workout ....see page 91.*
- *Intermediate Shoulder Workout ....see page 92.*
- *Advanced Shoulder Workout ....see page 93.*

Once you have progressed past these rehabilitative routines, you may want to attempt the following performance care routines:

- *Phase A – Getting Started with Shoulder Performance ....see page 96*
- *Phase B – Intermediate Shoulder Performance ....see page 97*
- *Phase C – Advanced Shoulder Performance ....see page 98*

If you currently have pain or inflammation in your shoulder, you may want to first reduce the inflammation with some of the following techniques:

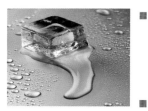

See "Cold Therapy" on page 186.

- **Apply cold packs**: A cold pack or ice can help if you have pain, swelling, or inflammation. Apply a cold pack to your shoulder for about 10 to15 minutes, two to three times a day.

- **Apply hot compresses**: Heat treatments should be used for chronic conditions to help relax and loosen tissues and to stimulate circulation to the area. Heat can help to increase oxygen levels, transport nutrients in, and transport waste products away.

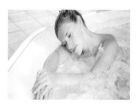

See "Heat Therapy" on page 188.

Apply a hot pack (or a cloth soaked in warm water) to the area where you feel the most pain or tenderness. Apply the hot pack for about 10 to15 minutes, two to three times a day. **Note:** Do not use hot compresses if there are any indications of inflammation, swelling, heat, or redness.

Warm-up for Your Shoulder

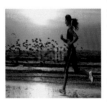

Review —> So what is a good warm-up?, page 43

Before starting any of our exercise routines, you need to perform a general cardiovascular warm-up that lasts approximately 10 to 15 minutes.

It doesn't matter if this is a brisk walk, a short jog, or riding a bicycle. (See *So what is a good warm-up? - page 43*.) The goal is to raise your body's core temperature enough to increase the elasticity of your muscles, tendons, ligaments, and joint structures. This cardiovascular workout will definitely speed your results and help to prevent any possible injuries that result from over-working cold, stiff muscles.

Once you have warmed up, you may want to do one or more of these warm-up massages before starting any neck exercise program to further relax and wake up your neck and shoulder muscles.

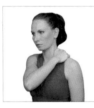

Massage Your Neck and Shoulders, page 119

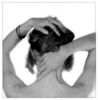

Massage the Back of Your Neck, page 120

Foam Roller for Your Shoulders, page 149

Beginner's Shoulder Workout

The exercises in the *Beginners Shoulder Workout* should always be performed in a completely **pain-free** state (as should any exercise in a rehabilitation protocol).

Before beginning this beginner's workout, take a few minutes to warm up and relax your body with the routines and massages shown in *Warm-up for Your Shoulder - page 90*.

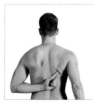

Setting and Activating the Scapulae, page 142

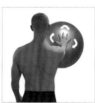

Ball Circles Against the Wall, page 144

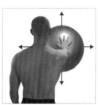

Four Cardinal Points with the Ball, page 145

Bringing in the Plane, page 143

Prone Y on the Floor, page 167

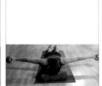

Prone T on the Floor, page 168

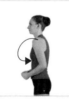

Shoulder Rolls, page 155

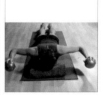

Prone L: Retract Your Scapulae, page 169

Beginner's Push-ups, page 157

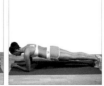

Beginner's Front Bridge, page 159

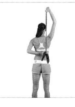

Triceps and Shoulder Stretch, page 147

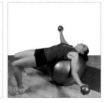

Ball Stretch for the Pectoralis, page 150

Intermediate Shoulder Workout

Before progressing to this workout, it is essential that you are able to comfortably perform the exercises in *Beginner's Shoulder Workout - page 91* for at least 1 to 2 weeks. Again, all the following exercise routines must be performed in a pain-free zone of safety.

For maximum benefit, before beginning this intermediate workout, take a few minutes to warm up your body (*So what is a good warm-up? - page 43*) and then relax the muscles of your shoulder with the routines and massages shown in *Warm-up for Your Shoulder - page 90.*

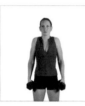
Stabilize and Strengthen Your Scapulae, page 170

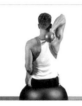
Lateral Raise with Tubing, page 162

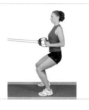
Standing Row with Tubing, page 172

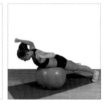
Swiss Ball Row, page 164

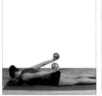
Shoulder Shrugs with Weights, page 154

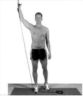
Work those Triceps and Shoulders, page 163

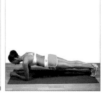
Beginner's Front Bridge, page 159

Intermediate Push-ups, page 158

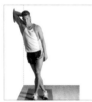
Leaning Into the Wall, page 148

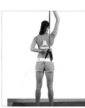
Triceps and Shoulder Stretch, page 147

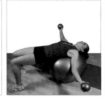
Ball Stretch for the Pectoralis, page 150

Foam Roller for Your Shoulders, page 149

Advanced Shoulder Workout

Before progressing to this **advanced** workout, it is essential that you are able to comfortably perform the exercises in *Intermediate Shoulder Workout - page 92*, for at least 1 to 2 weeks. Again, all the following exercise routines must be performed within a pain-free zone of safety.

For maximum benefit, before beginning this intermediate workout, take a few minutes to warm up your body (*So what is a good warm-up? - page 43*) and then relax the muscles of your shoulder with the routines and massages shown in *Warm-up for Your Shoulder - page 90*.

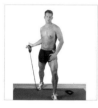

Throw a Javelin, page 165

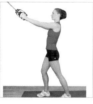

Strengthening the Latissimus Dorsi, page 173

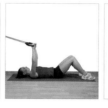

Chest Pull-Over with Tubing, page 175

Draw a Sword, page 166

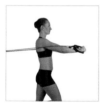

Chest Fly with Tubing, page 174

Prone Y on the Floor, page 167

Prone L: Retract Your Scapulae, page 169

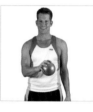

Lasso with a Handball, page 161

Push-ups with Unequal Hands, page 183

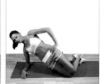

Beginner's Side Bridge – Knee Bent, page 160

Beginner's Four-Point Kneeling, page 176

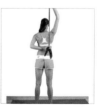

Triceps and Shoulder Stretch, page 147

Improving Your Shoulder's Athletic Performance

Improving your shoulder's performance is all about building power and strength from your core out to your extremities. It is about establishing strong, flexible links from the bottom of your feet, right up to your shoulders.

Shoulder performance training is also about increasing your ability to store and release energy. This ability is greatly dependent upon the quality of your soft tissues (muscles, ligaments, tendons, and connective tissue) and your capacity to recruit more of your nervous system.

Before you even consider doing these Performance routines, you must first have spent at least three weeks working on the Advanced Shoulder routines. You must also have been injury-free during that period of time.

Performance care is not like rehabilitative care. The demands on your body are much higher, but also allow you to achieve greater benefit. With these benefits come an increased risk of injury, especially if you are not ready for the training. To avoid possible injuries, make sure that you:

- Do perform an aerobic warm-up before any of these routines. Lack of proper warm-up is probably the most common cause of injury.
- Perform all the recommended stretches and myofascial work since they will help to build good quality tissue.
- Do *not* move up to the next level if you find that your muscles are not adapting to the demands you are placing on them. Stay at that level or move down by a level until your body adapts.
- Get some professional myofascial work done if your body is still not adapting, remains continually sore, or is very slow with recovery. Techniques such as *Active Release Techniques® (ART) - page 196* or *Massage Therapy - page 202* can get you back on your workout schedule.

A Workout for Increasing Shoulder Performance

The performance routines are divided into three main sections (A, B, C), each providing incrementally higher levels of difficulty. Each section prepares you for the next level by increasing the intensity of the routine. Many of these exercises make use of *unbalanced surfaces* or *altered positions* to recruit more of your nervous system for increased power development.

When you perform these exercises, it is extremely important to pay attention to your *eccentric contractions* (the return to your starting position). For example, in a push-up, take three to four counts to return to the starting position of a push-up (instead of just dropping to the ground). You will force your muscles to work much harder, and considerably speed your progress.

It is also essential to work on improving your core stability with any performance level routine. You will never develop true shoulder power and stability if you have a weak core. Development of core strength typically requires involvement of all the elements of your kinetic chain – from your legs and hips, through your core, and into your arms.

For maximum results, take the time to progress sequentially through all the levels of these performance care routines. The escalating difficulty within each phase helps you to pass each plateau, and move into the next level of performance. You will be working through the following levels:

- *Phase A – Getting Started with Shoulder Performance - page 96.*
- *Phase B – Intermediate Shoulder Performance - page 97.*
- *Phase C – Advanced Shoulder Performance - page 98.*

Performance routines use the '*super-set*' concept, where two or more exercises are performed consecutively, followed by a brief rest. Performing both exercises back-to-back is known as one *super-set*. As you advance through each phase, you will be performing multiple super-sets to help you increase performance.

Phase A - Getting Started with Shoulder Performance

Start with a 12-to-15 minute aerobic warm up. Then perform the following routines, using a tempo of 2–counts for the concentric contraction, and 2–counts for the eccentric contraction.

Super-set 1	Week 1 (1 set)	Week 2 (2 sets)	Week 3 (3 sets)
Prone Y on the Floor, page 167	10 reps	12 reps	14 reps
Front-to-Side Bridge, page 181	Hold for 5 seconds on each side.	Hold for 10 seconds on each side.	Hold for 15 seconds on each side.
REST FOR ONE MINUTE BEFORE NEXT SET or EXERCISE			

Super-set 2	Week 1 (1 set)	Week 2 (2 sets)	Week 3 (3 sets)
Prone T on the Floor, page 168	10 reps	12 reps	14 reps
Russian Twist with Medicine Ball, page 182	10 reps each side	12 reps each side	14 reps each side
REST FOR ONE MINUTE BEFORE NEXT SET or EXERCISE			

Super-set 3	Week 1 (1 set)	Week 2 (2 sets)	Week 3 (3 sets)
Advanced Four-Point Kneeling, page 177	10 reps	12 reps	14 reps
Chest Pull-Over with Tubing, page 175	10 reps	12 reps	14 reps
REST FOR ONE MINUTE BEFORE NEXT SET or EXERCISE			

End this routine with the stretching and myofascial release routines shown in *Stretching and Myofascial Exercises - page 99*.

Phase B - Intermediate Shoulder Performance

Start with a 12-to-15 minute aerobic warm up. Then perform the following routines, with a tempo of 2–counts for the concentric contraction, hold for 1–count, and 2–counts for the eccentric contraction.

Super-set 1	Week 1 (2 sets)	Week 2 (3 sets)	Week 3 (3 sets)
Prone L: Retract Your Scapulae, page 169	10 reps	12 reps	14 reps
Intermediate Push-ups, page 158	6-10 reps	8-12 reps	10-16 reps
REST FOR ONE MINUTE BEFORE NEXT SET or EXERCISE			

Super-set 2	Week 1 (2 sets)	Week 2 (3 sets)	Week 3 (3 sets)
Forward Bridge – Advanced, page 180	Hold for 10 seconds	Hold for 15 seconds	Hold for 20 seconds
Medicine Ball Wood Chop, page 178	10 reps each side	12 reps each side	14 reps each side
REST FOR ONE MINUTE BEFORE NEXT SET or EXERCISE			

Super-set 3	Week 1 (2 sets)	Week 2 (3 sets)	Week 3 (3 sets)
Prone Y on the Floor, page 167	10 reps	12 reps	14 reps
Strengthening the Latissimus Dorsi, page 173	10 reps	12 reps	14 reps
REST FOR ONE MINUTE BEFORE NEXT SET or EXERCISE			

End this routine with the stretching and myofascial release routines shown in *Stretching and Myofascial Exercises - page 99.*

Phase C - Advanced Shoulder Performance

Start with a 12-to-15 minute aerobic warm up. Then perform the following routines, with a tempo of 2–counts for the concentric contraction, hold for 1–count, and 3–counts for the eccentric contraction.

Super-set 1	Week 1 (2 sets)	Week 2 (3 sets)	Week 3 (3 sets)
Push-ups with Unequal Hands, page 183	6-8 reps	8-12 reps	10-16 reps
Prone Y on the Floor, page 167	10 reps	12 reps	14 reps
REST FOR ONE MINUTE BEFORE NEXT SET or EXERCISE			

Super-set 2	Week 1 (2 sets)	Week 2 (3 sets)	Week 3 (3 sets)
Prone T on the Floor, page 168	10 reps	12 reps	14 reps
Front-to-Side Bridge, page 181	Hold for 15 seconds on each side.	Hold for 20 seconds on each side.	Hold for 25 seconds on each side.
REST FOR ONE MINUTE BEFORE NEXT SET or EXERCISE			

Super-set 3	Week 1 (2 sets)	Week 2 (3 sets)	Week 3 (3 sets)
Prone L: Retract Your Scapulae, page 169	10 reps	12 reps	14 reps
Alternating Dumbbell Press on Ball, page 179	10 reps each hand	12 reps each hand	14 reps each hand
REST FOR ONE MINUTE BEFORE NEXT SET or EXERCISE			

End this routine with the stretching and myofascial release routines shown in *Stretching and Myofascial Exercises - page 99.*

Stretching and Myofascial Exercises

It is essential after each exercise session to incorporate myofascial work into your routines. This will speed your progress. prevent injury, and improve overall your ability to store and release energy.

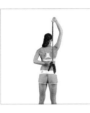

Triceps and
Shoulder Stretch,
page 147

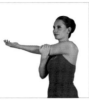

Arm-Across-Body
Stretch, page 150

Internal-External
Shoulder Stretch,
page 152

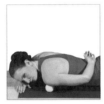

Tennis Ball –
Anterior Shoulder
Release, page 151

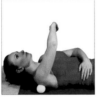

Tennis Ball –
Posterior Shoulder
Release, page 151

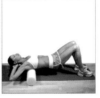

Foam Roller for
Your Shoulders,
page 149

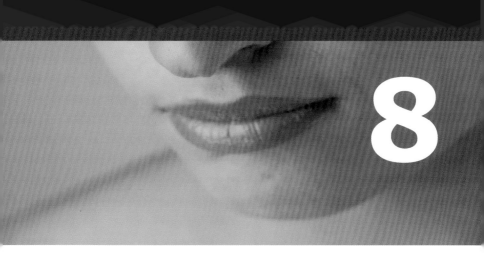

Exercises for the Jaw

Relaxing the Jaw

Strengthening and Stretching the Jaw

Pterygoid Massage - The lateral and medial pterygoid muscles are responsible for opening the jaw and depressing the mandible. These muscles also help in mastication (the process of chewing) and participate in performing the side-to-side and forward-back motions of the jaw. Tightness in these structures can prevent you from chewing properly.

It is very important to remove any restrictions in these muscles since there is a direct relationship between the muscles of your neck and jaw. Tension in the neck muscles will cause tension in the jaws, and vice-versa, tension in the muscles of the jaw will result in tension and stress in the muscles of the neck.

Use the following massage techniques to release the pterygoid muscles. There are several techniques that provide patients with similar exercises including Cyriax Orthapaedic Treatment Procedures, Applied Kinesiology, and Active Release Techniques.

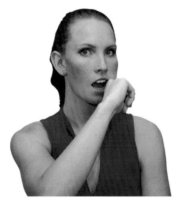 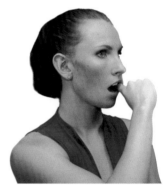

1. This is an **internal massage**, so wash your hands or use a rubber glove.
2. Open your mouth, and slide your finger along the upper teeth until you pass the last of the upper teeth, and are on the soft tissue at the back of your teeth.
3. Push the tip of your index finger back into the soft tissue.
    - Apply a moderate amount of pressure while gently kneading the area with the tip of your index finger. This area can be very sensitive.
    - Continue with this kneading motion for 30 to 45 seconds.
    - To reduce pain while performing this procedure, try slowly dropping your chin to your chest, and then slowly tilt your head to either side until you find a point where the pain is reduced.
4. Repeat this exercise for the opposite side of your jaw.
5. Do this exercise several times each day.

Temporal Massage - You can feel the temporalis muscles if you place your fingers on your temple, one inch behind your eyebrows, and then clench and unclench your teeth. This muscle acts to elevate and retract your mandibles – a large muscle that extends from your TM joint, up through your temples, and partly into your hairline. Massage of this area can relieve jaw pain since this muscle attaches to the TMJ.

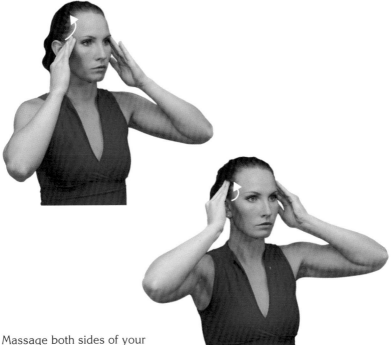

Massage both sides of your head at the same time:

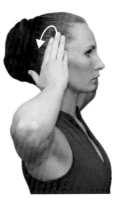

1. Using both hands, lightly place your fingertips just above the temporalis muscle as shown.

2. Start at the jaw's TMJ and use long strokes that extend up from the TMJ into your temples, and then around your ears to relax the muscle.

3. Repeat these strokes for about 60 seconds.

4. Now, apply gentle steady pressure on any points of tenderness (trigger points) until you feel a slight softening of the tension.

5. Repeat this exercise 3 times, several times a day.

Masseter Massage - The masseter is a large muscle that aids in raising the lower jaw and is used whenever you chew. Weakness and restrictions in the masseter can result in an inability to chew your food. To find your masseter, place your first two fingers on your jaw, just below your ears, and in-between your upper and lower molars. Then open and close your mouth, or clench your closed mouth to feel the masseters in operation.

This is a two-part massage, so wash your hands for the second part.

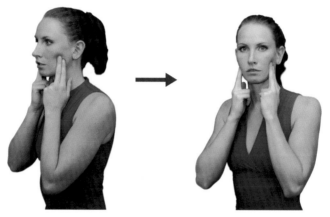

Part 1 – External Massage

1. Using either your fingertips or the heel of your palm, gently rub the jaw line of your face on both sides of your face.
   - Use small circular motions.
   - Work the area close to the end of the jaw (near your ear) to massage the masseter (the muscle used to open and close your jaw).

Part 2 – Internal Massage

1. This part is an internal massage, so wash your hands first. Use your right hand to massage your left masseter and vice-versa.

2. Open your mouth, and slide your *right* thumb along the *inside left* edge of your mouth until you find the masseter muscle.

3. Use your thumb (on the inside of your mouth) and your index finger (on the outside of your mouth) to pinch, massage, and rub the masseter muscle.
   - Every now and then, clench your jaw to ensure you are still working the masseter area.
   - Repeat these strokes for about 60 seconds.

4. Repeat the process for the opposite side.

5. Wash your hands when you have finished.

Activate Masseter Trigger Points - The masseter muscle is also responsible for the stabilization of the TMJ. This self-massage technique works on specific acupuncture points, and is very effective for reducing tension in the masseter muscles, increasing range of motion, and helping to eliminate trigger points in the tissues. Besides treating TMJ, this technique is also used in Traditional Chinese Medicine to relieve jaw spasms, reduce toothaches, facial pain, and treat Bell's Palsy.

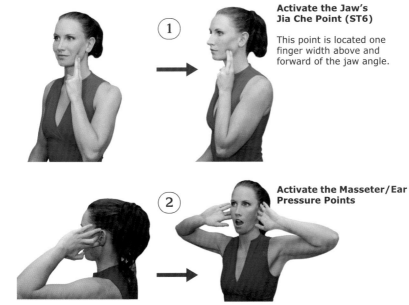

Activate the Jaw's Jia Che Point (ST6)

This point is located one finger width above and forward of the jaw angle.

Activate the Masseter/Ear Pressure Points

1. **Part 1: Activate the Jia Che Point (ST6).**
   - With two fingers, apply firm pressure to the point where the bottom of the masseter meets the outside corner of the jaw.
   - Hold this pressure for 30 seconds while performing small circular motions with your fingertips.
   - Repeat this exercise for the other side of your jaw.

2. **Part 2: Activate the Masseter/Ear Pressure Points.**
   - On both sides of your face, find the small hollow spot in front of the small triangular part of the ear with your middle finger. Open and close your jaw a few times to feel that small hollow.
   - Place a finger on the small hollow, a second finger where the top of your ear meets your head, and the third finger where the bottom of your ear meets your head.
   - Press *evenly* with all three fingers towards your skull.
   - Hold the pressure for 5 to 10 seconds.

3. Do this exercise several times each day.

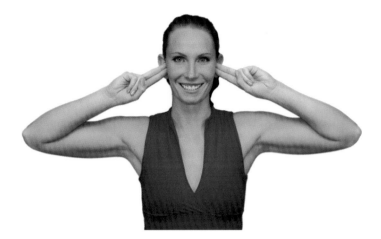

Strengthening and Stretching the Jaw

Functional Opening of the Jaw - In this exercise, you will be palpating and massaging the condylar head of your TMJ with your index finger. This exercise acts to increase circulation, jaw mobility, and motor/neuromuscular control. Restoration of this motor control is essential if you are suffering from a hyper-mobile joint.

Note: This exercise stimulates the Xia Guan (ST7) acupuncture point. This point is used to treat TMJ, facial pain, and upper jaw toothaches.

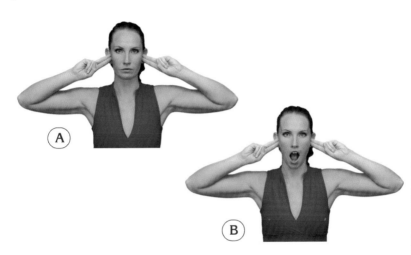

S1	10R
S2	8R
S3	6R

1. **Stimulate the Xia Guan point (ST7)**
   - Keep your tongue pressed against the hard palate of your mouth, with the tip just behind your front teeth. This position will give you feedback about your TMJ motion.
   - Place your forefingers by your ears as shown in image A.
   - Use your index fingers to locate the condylar head of your TMJ at the back of your mouth. It will feel like a small indentation when your mouth is open.

2. Keep your finger in this indentation and apply moderate pressure directly towards your skull.

3. Slowly *open* and *close* your jaw while limiting any jaw deviations, and always working within your pain-free zone.

4. Repeat this exercise for the recommended number of sets and repetitions.

Assisted Opening of the Mouth - TMJ, with its accompanying tightening of the jaw muscles, often makes it difficult to open and close your mouth. In this exercise, you will use your hand to gently assist your mouth in opening and closing.

Do not use a lot of force! You should not feel any pain when you do this exercise. Exercising while you are in pain creates abnormal motor control patterns that you do not want to reinforce. To truly rehabilitate your injuries, you must work within a pain-free zone.

S1
6R

S2
4R

S3
2R

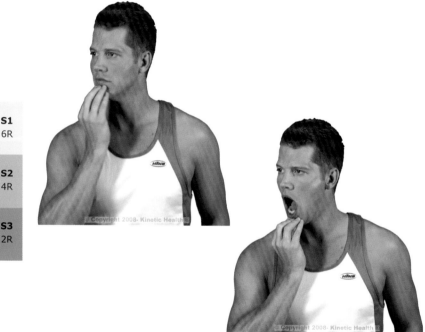

1. Place your fingertips gently just below your lips.
2. Slowly open your mouth as wide as you comfortably can.
3. Use your hand and pull gently downwards to open the mouth just a little more.
4. Hold this stretch for 4 to 5 seconds.
5. Now *slowly* close your mouth.
6. Repeat this exercise for the recommended number of sets and repetitions.

Resisted Opening of the Mouth - This resistance exercise helps to increase the strength of your jaw muscles. Again, take your time, be gentle, and stop if you feel pain.

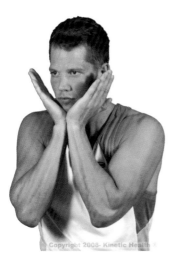

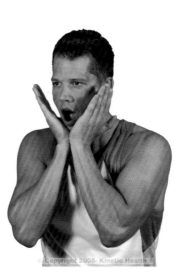

S1
6R

S2
4R

S3
2R

1. Place the palms of both hands just below your chin as shown above.
2. Slowly open your mouth as wide as you comfortably can, and at the same time push gently upwards (as if to prevent your mouth from opening).
3. Hold the open-mouth resistance for 5 seconds.
4. Now *slowly* close your mouth while maintaining moderate resistance with the palm of your hands.
5. Repeat this exercise for the recommended number of sets and repetitions.

Protracting and Retracting the Jaw - The goal of this exercise is to increase the mobility of your lower jaw, especially its forward/back motions. This important action affects your ability to chew food. Use this exercise if you suffer from TMJ pain or have jaw alignment problems.

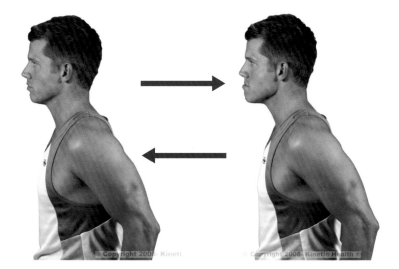

S1
8R

S2
6R

S3
4R

1. Start with your spine in neutral position, ears aligned over your shoulder, with your shoulders back (not rolled forward), and your scapula retracted.
2. Place the palms of your hand against your lower back to help maintain the correct posture.
3. Keeping your lips sealed, place the tip of your tongue on the roof of your mouth, and push your lower jaw forward in a jutting action.
4. Hold the protracted position of your jaw for three seconds.
5. Return to the starting position, and repeat the exercise for the recommended number of sets and repetitions.

Lateral Mobilization of the Jaw - Many people who suffer from jaw pain will notice that their jaw deviates more to one side than the other. This exercise helps you to maintain lateral jaw symmetry and balances the muscles on both sides of the jaw. It must be performed within a pain-free range of motion.

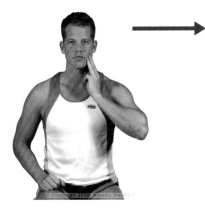
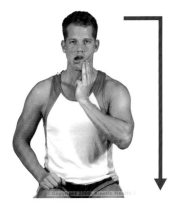
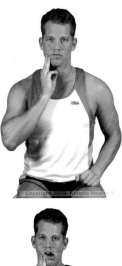

S1
6R

S2
4R

S3
2R

1. Start with your spine in neutral position, ears aligned over your shoulders.

2. Relax your jaw muscles.

3. Using the fingers of your left hand, gently push your lower jaw to the right.

4. Hold that position for eight seconds.

5. Let your jaw return to its neutral position.

6. Repeat the procedure for the right side, using your right hand to gently push your jaw to the left side.

7. Repeat this sequence for the recommended number of sets and reps for *both* sides of your jaw.

Fist in Mouth... Stretching the TMJ - Many people who suffer from TMJ syndromes cannot open their mouth properly. This exercise may seem unsanitary initially, but it really works, and can help you to relax all the muscles of your jaw as well as increase the range of motion of your TMJ.

Note: Wash your hands well before starting this exercise, and of course, when you have finished the exercise!

S1
5R

S2
4R

S3
3R

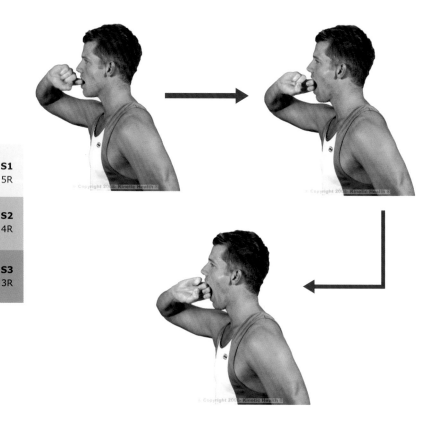

1. Open your mouth and place the knuckle of one finger between your lips.
2. If you are able to open your mouth comfortably, try placing the knuckles of your two fingers between your lips.
3. Once you are able to do step 2 comfortably, open your mouth even wider, and try to place the knuckles of three fingers between your lips.
4. In each step, hold your mouth open for at least 1 to 15 seconds.
5. Repeat this exercise for the recommended numbers of sets and reps, several times a day.

Clicking Your Tongue - A common issue with jaw and TMJ
problems is the movement of the jaw and tongue away from their normal neutral, resting position.

The tongue-clicking exercise (funny as it sounds) helps to return your jaw back into its resting position and restores normal nasal and diaphragmatic breathing. Once you are able to establish this alignment, you should continue to keep your tongue in this neutral position (tongue positioned against your hard palate) as you go about your daily living activities.

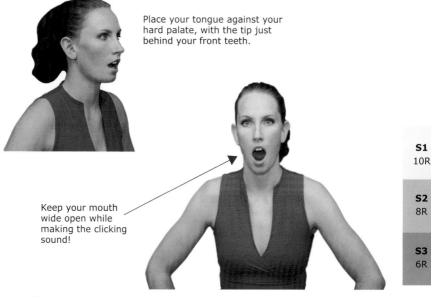

Place your tongue against your hard palate, with the tip just behind your front teeth.

Keep your mouth wide open while making the clicking sound!

S1
10R

S2
8R

S3
6R

1.   Place your tongue against the hard palate, with the tip of your tongue resting just behind your front teeth.

2.   With your mouth wide open, make a **clicking** sound with your tongue by quickly releasing its contact with your hard palate.

3.   Repeat this exercise for the recommended number of sets and reps.

Note: During your normal working day, become aware of the position of your jaw and tongue. In its normal resting position, the tongue should be in contact with the hard palate. This position lets you perform your normal nasal and diaphragmatic breathing.

Isometric Jaw Resistance - In this exercise you will apply resistance to the actions of closing, opening, and lateral deviation of your jaw while it is in a resting position. There should be no movement of your jaw while doing this exercise. The goal of this exercise is to establish normal alignment of the jaw while maintaining its correct postural position.

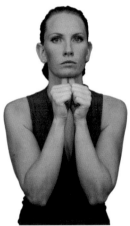

Resisted Jaw Opening 1

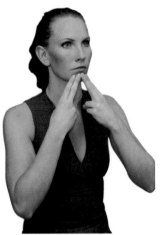

Resisted Jaw Opening 2

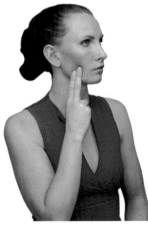

Resisted Lateral Motion

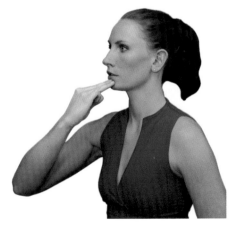

Resisted Jaw Protrusion

Isometric Jaw Resistance Exercises (continued) - All of the following steps should be performed in a pain-free state. If you start to feel pain, you are using too much pressure. Back off, and try again.

1. Start with your mouth closed, and your tongue resting against your hard palate, with the tip just behind your front teeth.

2. **Resisted Jaw Opening 1:**
   - Place your thumbs under your chin to keep your jaw from moving.
   - Attempt to open your mouth, but use your thumbs to resist this motion.
   - Hold for a count of 5.

3. **Resisted Jaw Opening 2:**
   - Place your fingertips at your chin, just below your lips, and press gently to keep your jaw from moving.
   - Attempt to open your mouth with a downward pressure of your fingers.
   - **Resist** this motion with your jaw muscles.
   - Do not allow your mouth to open.
   - Hold for a count of 5.

   S1
   5 sec

4. **Resisted Lateral Motion:**
   Do the following for **both** sides of your face.
   - Place your first two fingers against your lower teeth and push gently to move the jaw to the opposite side.
   - **Resist** this motion with your jaw muscles. Do not allow your mouth to open.
   - Hold for a count of 5.

   S2
   5 sec

   S3
   5 sec

5. **Resisted Jaw Protrusion:**
   - Place your fingertips at your chin, just below your lips.
   - Press gently to keep your jaw from moving.
   - Push your jaw forward gently, without opening your mouth.
   - **Resist** this motion with your fingertips. Do not allow your mouth to open.
   - Hold for a count of 5.

TMJ Opening and Closing - A common TMJ problem is excessive hyper-mobility when chewing or masticating food. The mastication process requires a combination of hinge and rotational movement by the joints of your jaw.

This exercise trains your jaw so that you can prevent excessive jaw protrusion, while still allowing for the required rotational movements. You can even use this exercise to reduce jaw hyper-mobility while you eat! This is a key exercise for "**grooving**" motor control patterns.

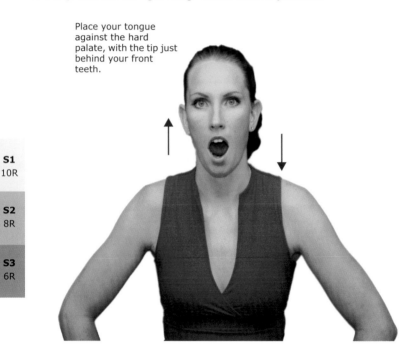

Place your tongue against the hard palate, with the tip just behind your front teeth.

S1
10R

S2
8R

S3
6R

1. Place your tongue against the hard palate, with the tip just behind your front teeth.
2. Keeping your tongue touching the hard palate, open and close your mouth slightly. Stay within a pain-free range of motion.
3. Repeat this exercise for the recommended number of sets and reps.

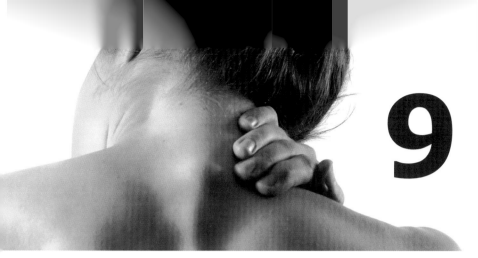

Exercises for the Neck

Relaxing the Neck

Stretching the Neck

Strengthening the Neck

Massage Your Neck and Shoulders - Massage (including self-massage) is the ideal way to relax those tense neck and shoulder muscles that we all have.

Try the following self-massage tips to warm-up and loosen those tight neck areas before beginning any neck exercise routine. Be sure to use some oil or cream if you are massaging directly on bare skin.

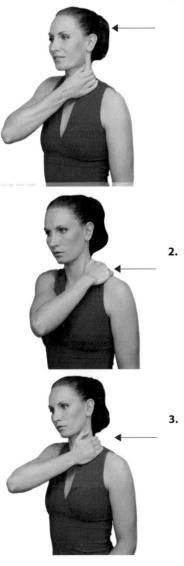

1. **Squeeze and release the sides of your neck:**
   - With the fingers of one hand, reach across to the opposite side of your neck, near the base of your skull.
   - Gently squeeze and release, working along the side of the neck and down the arm to the elbow.
   - Glide back to your neck and repeat at least 3 times for each side.
   - **Note**: Do not massage the front of your neck as there are important arteries and veins that you need to stay away from.

2. **Stroke the outer curve of your shoulder:**
   - Wrap your hand around the base of your neck, fingertips touching your spine.
   - Firmly stroke from the back of your shoulders to the front in a smooth continuous motion.
   - Glide back to your neck and repeat at least 3 times for each side.

3. **Massage your muscles around your spine:**
   - Use your fingertips to make small circular motions around either side of your spine.
   - Work from just below your shoulders to the base of your skull.

Massage the Back of Your Neck - Use the following techniques to relax and wake up the muscles and nerves of your face, neck, and shoulders. You should feel a substantial difference between the side that you have worked, and the side that you have not massaged.

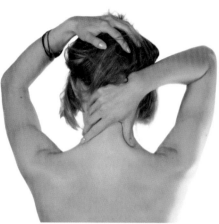

1. Use your thumb and index finger to knead the tension out from your lower to mid- neck.

2. Use gentle circular motions once you reach the base of your skull. This is the insertion point for many of your neck muscles, and a frequent point of tension.

Release Your Sinuses - This massage releases tension and fluid build-up from your sinuses and temples.

1. With the tips of your fingers, apply small circular motions over the areas shown in this image.

   Each of these areas lies directly over one of your sinuses, and some also correspond to acupuncture points.

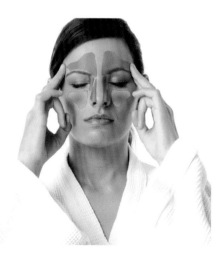

Foam Roller for Your Neck - When your neck and shoulder muscles are really tight, you will be amazed at how quickly they relax with the following foam roller exercise. This exercise releases tightness in the upper neck (suboccipital and neck extensors), as well as in the lower neck (levator scapulae, upper trapezius, splenius capitis, and semispinalis capitis muscles).

CAUTION: **Never** use the foam roller along the front or sides of your neck. Several critical arteries and veins (including the carotid artery) pump blood from your heart to your head and back. Crushing these with a foam roller could result in serious injury.

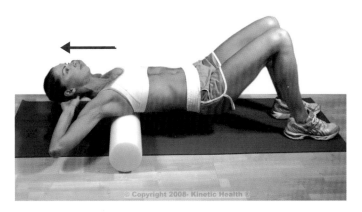

1. Lie on your back so that the foam roller is perpendicular to your spine, and placed just under your shoulder.

    ■ Bend your knees and place your feet flat on the ground.
    ■ Brace your core and lift your hips off the ground so that your body forms a straight line.

2. Roll back and forth on the foam roller, from the top of your shoulders to the base of your skull. **DO NOT** roll onto the sides or front of your neck since you could crush delicate veins and arteries.

3. Repeat this action 5 to10 times.

Stretching the Neck

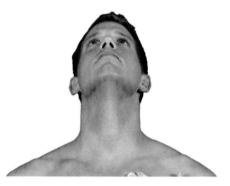

Perform these neck stretches after you have done your cardiovascular warm-up, and remember to breathe while holding the stretch for the recommended period of time. Don't bounce during any of these stretches, as bouncing can result in increased muscle tension, which could cause the formation of more restrictions. These exercise must be performed within a pain-free range of motion to avoid creating abnormal motor responses. If you feel pain, then you are stretching too far, and need to back off to the point where there is no pain!

❏ Shoulder Check ....see page 123

❏ Ears to your Shoulder ....see page 124

❏ See your Shoes, Watch the Stars ....see page 125

❏ Make Like a Rooster ....see page 126

❏ Get that Double Chin ....see page 127

❏ Stretch Your Upper Back ....see page 128

Note: Do not perform these stretches if you are in a period of acute muscle strain, have fractured the area, or have a joint injury in the neck/shoulder region. Give your muscles a chance to rest, and then return to these stretches once you are past the acute phase.

Shoulder Check - This exercise assists in developing lateral cervical rotation of the neck and head. You use this motion whenever you perform a shoulder check when driving. This exercise focuses not only on increasing your active range of motion but also helps to establish normal neurological motor patterns. Again, this exercise must be performed within a pain-free range of motion to avoid creating abnormal motor responses.

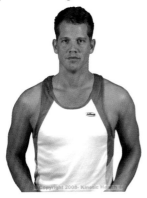

1. Sit or stand, with your spine in neutral position, head up, and ears aligned over your shoulders. Inhale deeply.

2. Gently stretch your head as far to the right as you can.
   - Exhale as you carry out this stretch.
   - Stop when you feel the stretch on the left side of your neck.
   - Hold this extended position for at least five seconds, while breathing normally.

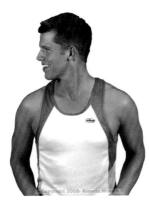

3. Return to your starting position. Inhale deeply.

4. Now turn your head as far to the left as you can.
   - Exhale as you carry out this stretch.
   - Stop when you feel the stretch on the right side of your neck.
   - Hold this extended position for at least 15 to 20 seconds, while breathing normally.

5. Repeat this exercise 5 to 10 times for each side.

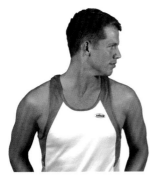

Ears to your Shoulder - This exercise focuses on increasing your active range of motion for lateral flexion and establishes normal neurological motor patterns (or **grooving**). The process of grooving motor responses is very important for developing power in your neck. Power is a function of how efficiently you can recruit your nervous system to synchronize the activation of muscles. The more efficient this system is, the more power you will have, and the fewer the number of injuries.

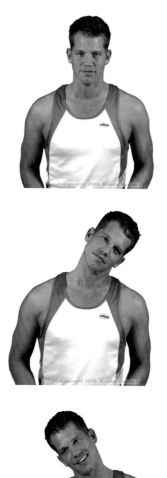

1. Sit or stand, with your spine in neutral position, head up, and ears aligned over your shoulders. Inhale deeply.

2. Exhale and gently bend your neck to the right side, as if you are trying to touch your ear to your shoulder.
   - Do not shrug or raise your shoulders.
   - Hold this extended position for five seconds, while breathing normally.

3. Return to your starting position. Inhale deeply.

4. Now exhale and gently bend your neck to the left side, as if you are trying to touch your ear to your shoulder.

5. Hold this extended position for 10 to 15 seconds, while breathing normally.

6. Repeat this exercise 5 to 10 times for each side.

See your Shoes, Watch the Stars - This is a flexion-extension exercise for the muscles in the front and back of your neck. This exercise is great for reducing and preventing neck pain and for increasing neck stability. It stretches and strengthens the muscles in the back of your head, as well as the neck flexors in the front of your neck. It is useful for reducing symptoms from conditions such as chronic neck pain, whiplash injuries, anterior (forward) posture syndromes, and headaches.

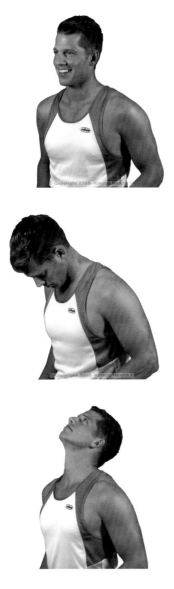

1. Sit or stand, with your spine in neutral position, head up, and ears aligned over your shoulders. Inhale deeply.

2. Gently tip your head forward as far as you can.
   - Exhale as you perform this stretch.
   - Try to see your toes. You should feel the stretch on the back of your neck.
   - Hold this position for 5 to 10 seconds, while breathing normally.

3. Return to your starting position. Inhale deeply.

4. Now tip your head backward as far as you can.
   - Exhale as you perform this stretch.
   - You should be looking at the top of the ceiling (or sky, if you are outside!)
   - Hold this position for 5 to 10 seconds, while breathing normally.

5. Repeat this sequence 5 to 10 times.

Make Like a Rooster - This neck protraction/retraction exercise stretches and strengthens the postural muscles in the back and front of your neck. Doing this exercise on a regular basis can help you to correct the results of a slouching, head-forward posture, and reduce symptoms from conditions such as Thoracic Outlet Syndrome and TMJ dysfunctions.

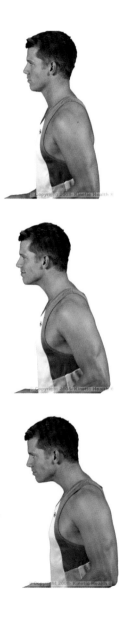

1. Sit or stand, with your spine in neutral position, head up, and ears aligned over your shoulders. Inhale deeply.

2. Exhale, and gently push your neck forward (like a rooster).
   - You should feel your head glide forward on your spine.
   - Hold this position for five seconds, while breathing normally.

3. Return to your starting position.

4. Inhale deeply and repeat this stretch 5 to 10 times.

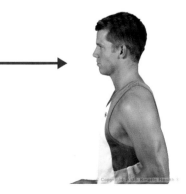

Get that Double Chin - This chin protraction/retraction exercise stretches and strengthens the postural muscles in the back and front of your neck. Doing this exercise on a regular basis can help you to correct the results of a slouching, head-forward posture, and reduce symptoms resulting from conditions such as Thoracic Outlet Syndrome and TMJ dysfunctions.

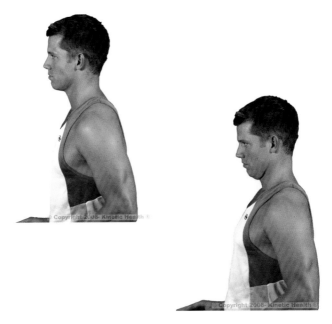

1. Sit or stand, with your spine in neutral position, head up, and ears aligned over your shoulders. Inhale deeply.

2. Exhale, and gently pull your neck backward.
   - You should feel your head glide back on to your spine.
   - Did you make a double chin?
   - Hold this position for 10 to 15 seconds, while breathing normally.

3. Return to your starting position. Inhale deeply and repeat this stretch another 5 to 10 times.

Note: If you have difficulty performing step 2, try this variation. Put your finger on your chin, exhale, and gently press your chin back. Everything else is the same as above.

Stretch Your Upper Back - The upper back can often be an awkward area to stretch since it contains many different layers of muscles. This exercise is great for stretching out these layers, including your trapezius, rhomboids, and cervical and upper thoracic paraspinals. You will need a fitness ball for this exercise.

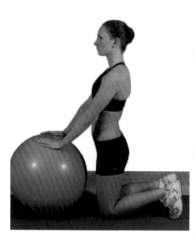

1. Starting Position:
   - Kneel on the floor on all fours.
   - Place both hands on top of the fitness ball.

2. Push the ball out in front of you with both arms.
   - Ensure your torso and head are aligned, face down towards the floor.
   - Inhale.

3. Exhale, drop your head between your shoulders, and:
   - Arch your back.
   - Sit back on your heels.
   - Maintain your hold on the ball.

4. Hold this stretch for 30 to 60 seconds.
   - You should feel the stretch between your scapula, through your arms, and down your spine.

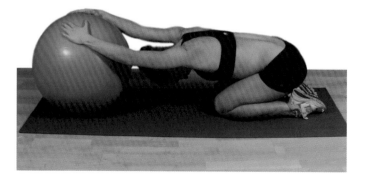

Strengthening the Neck

Benefits of PNF Exercises

PNF, or Proprioceptive Neuromuscular Facilitation, is a form of flexibility training that combines the contracting of specific muscle groups with stretching to increase the active range of motion (ROM).

PNF is an advanced form of stretching that targets specific muscle groups. It results in substantial increases in flexibility, with an accompanying increase in muscle strength. Originally, PNF exercises were developed to help stroke victims recover and rehabilitate their muscles.

PNF stretching takes advantage of the sudden increase in elasticity of the muscle (which only lasts for a short time after an isometric contraction) to increase the range of motion. During a PNF exercise, it is very important to EXHALE **after** an *isometric contraction* (a static muscle contraction that occurs *without* movement).

You can make substantial gains in soft tissue flexibility by using PNF exercises. PNF is acknowledged as being one of the fastest, and most effective means for increasing passive, static flexibility.

Attention: PNF stretches are only recommended for intermediate to advanced users. You should first be able to perform all the Beginner-level stretches comfortably before attempting PNF stretches. Also...PNF stretches should *not* be done more than 3 times per week.

Isometric Neck Resistance - With this exercise, you will apply resistance to the flexion and extension of your neck while it maintains a neutral position. (See the next page for step-by-step instructions).

There should be **no movement of your neck** while doing these exercises, and all motions should be performed in a **pain-free** zone. The goal of this exercise is to establish normal alignment of the neck while maintaining its neutral postural position.

S1
5R

S2
4R

S3
3R

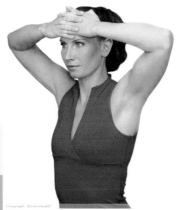

Resisting Neck Flexion

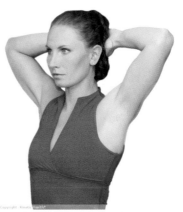

Resisting Neck Extension

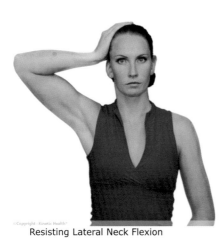

Resisting Lateral Neck Flexion

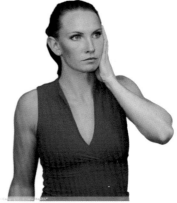

Resisting Neck Rotation

Isometric Neck Resistance Exercises (continued)

See the images on the facing page for examples of each exercise.

1. For each of the following exercises, ensure that you sit or stand, with your back straight, head up, ears aligned over your shoulders.

2. **Resisting Neck Flexion**: There should be **no movement of your neck**, and **no pain** when you do this exercise.
   - Place the palm of your hands flat on your forehead.
   - Firmly push your forehead forward against the palm of your hands.
   - Apply resistive pressure for 5 to 8 seconds and slowly release.

3. **Resisting Neck Extension**: There should be **no movement of your neck**, and **no pain** when you do this exercise.
   - Clasp your hands behind your head.
   - Firmly push the back of your head against your hands.
   - Apply resistive pressure for 5 to 8 seconds and release.

4. **Resisting Lateral Neck Flexion**: There should be **no movement of your neck**, and **no pain** when you do this exercise.
   - Place palm of your hand above your left ear, and wrap your fingers around the top of your head.
   - Firmly push the top of your head against your hand while fully resisting the motion with your left hand.
   - Apply resistive pressure for 5 to 8 seconds and release.
   - Repeat this procedure for your right side.

5. **Resisting Neck Rotation**: There should be **no movement of your neck**, and **no pain** when you do this exercise.
   - Place palm of your right hand against the right side of your face.
   - Firmly push the side of your face against your hand, while fully resisting the motion with your right hand.
   - Apply resistive pressure for 5 to 8 seconds and release.
   - Repeat this procedure for your left side.

Repeat this series of exercise for the recommended number of sets and repetitions**.**

PNF – Extend Your Neck and Head - This cervical flexion-extension exercise works the muscles in the front and back of your neck. This exercise is great for reducing and preventing neck pain, and for increasing neck stability. It strengthens the extensor muscles in the back of your head, as well as stretches the neck flexors in the front of your neck. It is useful for reducing symptoms from conditions such as neck pain, whiplash, thoracic outlet syndrome, and for correcting the results of a slouching, head-forward posture.

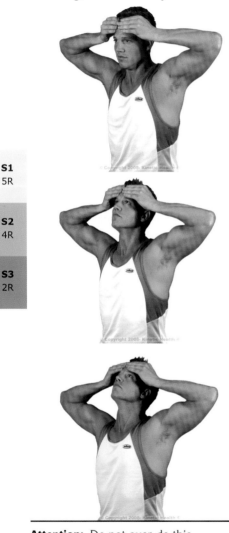

S1
5R

S2
4R

S3
2R

1. Sit or stand, with your spine in neutral position, head up, and ears aligned over your shoulders. Inhale deeply.

2. Place your fingers on your forehead and inhale deeply.

3. Exhale and press your head forward into your hands.
   - Use both hands to resist this head motion for 5 to 8 seconds.
   - Do not allow your head to move forward.

4. Inhale deeply as you release all tension and extend your head further back, to about one-third of its maximum extension range.

5. Repeat Step 3 again from this new position.

6. Inhale deeply and release all tension as you tip your head back to about two-thirds of its maximum extension range.

7. Repeat Step 3 again from this new position.

8. Finally, inhale deeply as you release all tension, and extend your head as far back as you can. You should be able to extend back farther than you could before.

9. Repeat this entire sequence for the recommended number of sets and repetitions.

Attention: Do not over-do this exercise.

PNF – Flex Your Neck and Head

PNF – Flex Your Neck and Head - This flexion-extension exercise for the muscles in the front and back of your neck is great for reducing and preventing neck pain, and for increasing neck stability. It stretches the extensor muscles in the back of your head, as well as strengthens the neck flexors in front of your neck. It is useful for reducing symptoms from conditions such as whiplash, neck pain, thoracic outlet syndrome, and for correcting the results of a slouching, head-forward posture.

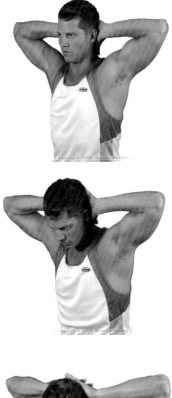

1. Sit or stand, with your spine in neutral position, head up, and ears aligned over your shoulders. Inhale deeply.

2. Lock your hands behind the base of your skull.

3. Exhale, and press your head backward into your hands.
   - Use both hands to resist this head motion for 5 to 8 seconds.
   - Do not allow your head to move backward.

   S1
   5R

4. Inhale deeply as you release all tension and flex your head forward, to about one-third of its maximum flexion range for 5 to 8 seconds.

   S2
   4R

5. Repeat Step 3 again from this new position.

   S3
   3R

6. Inhale deeply and release all tension as you move your head to two-thirds of its maximum flexion range for 5 to 8 seconds.

7. Repeat Step 3 again from this new position.

8. Finally, inhale deeply as you release all your tension and flex forward as far as you can for 5 to 8 seconds. You should be able to flex farther forward than you could before.

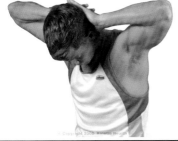

9. Repeat this entire sequence for the recommended number of sets and repetitions.

Attention: Do not over-do this exercise.

PNF – Laterally Flex Your Neck and Head - This exercise focuses on stretching and strengthening the muscles on the sides of your neck (lateral flexion). Doing this exercise regularly will help increase flexibility to the neck and shoulders, and prevent conditions such as neck pain and thoracic outlet syndrome. Use this exercise to stretch the scalenes and trapezius muscles.

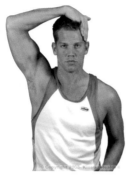

1. Sit or stand, with your spine in neutral position, head up, and ears aligned over your shoulders. Inhale deeply.

2. Take your right hand, and wrap it over the top of your head, with your fingertips just above your left ear. Inhale deeply.

3. Exhale, and push your head towards the left side, so that you are pushing your head into your right hand, towards your shoulder.

    ■ Resist this head motion with your hand for 4 seconds.

4. Inhale deeply as you release all tension and laterally flex your head further towards your right arm, to about half of its maximum flexion range, and hold for 5 to 8 seconds.

5. Repeat Step 3 from this new position.

S1
5R

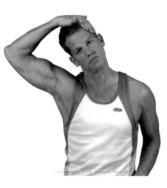

S2
4R

S3
3R

6. Finally, inhale deeply as you release all your tension and laterally flex your head as far to the right as you can. You should be able to laterally flex farther than you could before.

7. Repeat this exercise for the recommended number of sets and repetitions for **each** side.

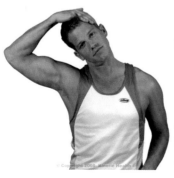

Note: You should feel a comfortable stretch, without pain. The scalenes can be a sensitive area to stretch.

PNF – Cervical Rotation of Your Head -

This cervical rotation exercise focuses on stretching and strengthening the lateral rotation muscles of your neck. You use this motion whenever you perform a shoulder check when driving, and for many other daily activities.

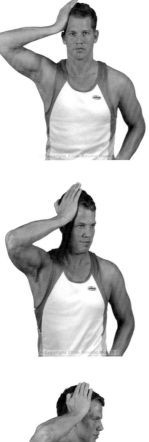

1. Sit or stand, with your spine in neutral position, head up, and ears aligned over your shoulders. Inhale deeply.

2. Place the heel of your right hand on your right temple above your ear. Inhale deeply.

3. Exhale, and turn your head to the **left**.

4. Now, push your head into your *right* hand, and resist this head motion with your right hand for 5 to 8 seconds.

5. Inhale deeply as you release all tension and rotate your head further to the left, to about half of its rotational range and hold for 4 seconds.

6. Now push your head back into your right hand.
   - Apply just enough resistance to keep the head static.
   - Hold the resistance position for 5 to 8 seconds, while breathing normally.

7. Inhale deeply as you release all the tension and rotate your head as far as you can to the *left*. You should be able to rotate your head farther than you could before.

8. Repeat this exercise for the recommended number of sets and repetitions for **each** side.

S1	5R
S2	4R
S3	3R

Attention: Do not over-do this exercise.

PNF – Stretch your Levator Scapulae - This exercise focuses on increasing the strength and flexibility of your neck and the muscles that attach to your shoulder blade (scapula) and lower cervical spine.

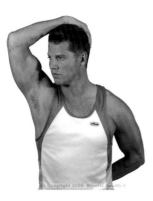

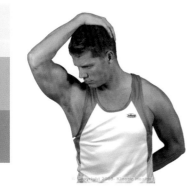

S1
5R

S2
4R

S3
3R

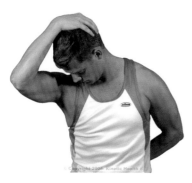

1. Sit or stand, with your spine in neutral position, head up, and face turned right to a 45 degree angle.

2. Take your right hand, and wrap it over the top of your head.

3. Push your head back against the palm of your right hand for a count of 5 to 8 seconds. Inhale.

4. Exhale deeply, and slowly lower your head diagonally downwards for a count of 4 seconds.

5. Use your hand to hold your head in that position, and push your head **back** into your hands.

   ■ Hold the position for a count of 5 to 8 seconds seconds.

   ■ Apply just enough resistance to keep the head static.

6. Now relax, and inhale.

7. Exhale and slowly lower your head diagonally forward (as far as it will comfortably go) for another count of 4 seconds.

8. Repeat this exercise for the recommended number of sets and repetitions, for **both** sides of your neck.

Attention: Do not over-do this exercise.

Strengthen Your Neck with a Swiss Ball - Use this exercise to strengthen the muscles of your neck, while activating your core and enhancing your balance and proprioception.

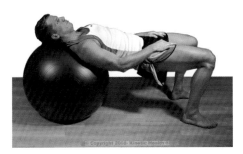

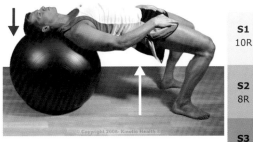

S1
10R

S2
8R

S3
6R

1. Achieve the following starting position.

    ■ Sit on the ball, with your hands by your side.
    ■ Walk your feet out, rolling your hips down and lying back on the ball as you do this.
    ■ Stop when your neck and shoulder blades are resting on the ball.
    ■ Lower your head onto the ball.
    ■ Contract your gluteals and raise your hips so your body is parallel to the ground, as shown above.
    ■ Brace your core.

2. Press your head down for a count of 5, and then release.

3. Repeat this exercise for the recommended number of sets and repetitions.

Attention: Make sure you brace your abdominals and gluteals when doing this exercise. See *How to Brace your Core! - page 15* for more information.

Cat-Camel Stretch - The flexion and extension motion of the spine that occurs during this exercise creates a pumping action which acts to displace fluid collecting in the discs of your vertebrae. Do this exercise as soon as you wake up every morning.

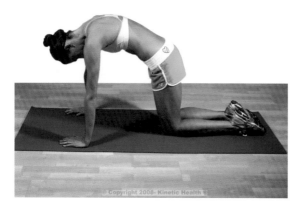

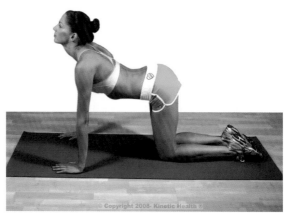

1. Kneel on the floor, with your hands and feet shoulder-width apart, palms flat on the ground.

2. Slowly move into the camel stretch by curving your spine and dropping your head down between your shoulders.

3. Now move into the cat stretch by arching your back towards the ground and raising your chin up towards the ceiling. Your buttocks should rise into the air.

4. Move back and forth between the Camel and Cat stretches, 15 to 20 times, to pump the excess fluid out of your discs.

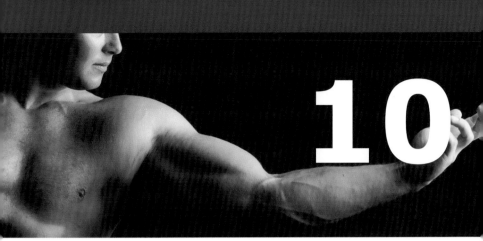

10

Exercises for the Shoulder

Body Awareness for the Shoulder

Stretches for the Shoulder

Strengthening the Shoulder

Beginner

Performance Care Exercises for the Shoulder

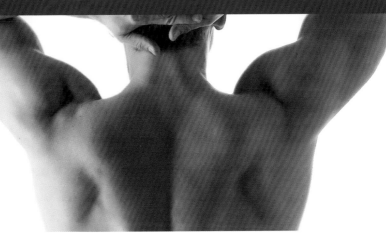

Body Awareness for the Shoulder

Performing the following exercises helps you to become more aware of the structures in your shoulder and in its kinetic chain. The shoulder joint is capable of complex motions and consists of many inter-related layers of muscle and soft tissue.

Due to this complexity, it is important to take a few minutes to become aware of these structures. In addition, the full impact of these exercises will not be realized unless you *maintain proper shoulder alignment.*

The following exercises help you to become aware of the correct positioning of your shoulder, and help to ensure that you are able to achieve the full benefit of the subsequent shoulder exercises.

❏ Setting and Activating the Scapulae ....see page 142

❏ Bringing in the Plane ....see page 143

❏ Ball Circles Against the Wall ....see page 144

❏ Four Cardinal Points with the Ball ....see page 145

Setting and Activating the Scapulae - Start every upper body
exercise with your shoulders in the position shown here. This exercise helps
you to build awareness of where the scapula is and learn what its normal
positioning should be. You will need this awareness to do the remainder of
the exercises in this chapter. Always start with this exercise.

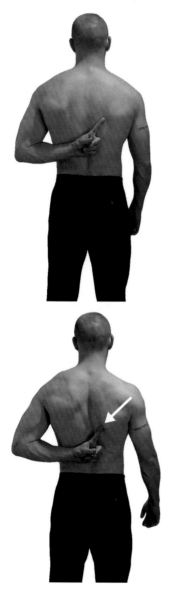

1. Stand straight, with both hands hanging loosely by your sides.

2. Extend the forefinger of your left hand and reach behind your back to lightly touch the medial (bottom inner) edge of your right scapula or shoulder blade. Keep the other arm relaxed.

3. Bring both scapulae downwards and towards the midline of your back to activate the lower trapezius muscles. You should be pushing towards the finger that is touching the scapula.

    ■ Ensure you do not activate any other muscles.

    ■ Keep the upper trapezius and latissimus dorsi of your back relaxed.

    ■ The entire movement should come from the muscles (lower trapezius) pushing the scapula down onto the finger.

    ■ This is the scapula's *normal* (and desired) position, where the bottom of the scapula has flattened out.

    ■ Conduct most of the exercises in this chapter with you scapulae in this position.

4. Hold this position for 3 to 5 seconds and then take 3 to 5 seconds to slowly release and return to neutral position. Repeat 3 to 5 times on each side.

Note: Bad scapular positioning will cause the bottom edge of the scapula to protrude outwards.

Bringing in the Plane - This exercise helps you to activate and build awareness of your lower trapezius muscle, which contributes both strength and stability to the shoulders. It is essential to activate and control the lower trapezius in order to reduce chances of injury and to ensure proper recovery from shoulder injuries.

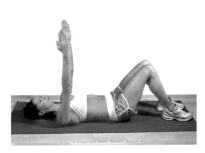

Do this exercise before beginning the balance of the Shoulder exercise program.

1. Lie flat on your back and reset your scapulae to the normal position as described in *Setting and Activating the Scapulae - page 142.*

2. Raise your arms so that they are perpendicular to the ground.

3. **Very slowly** lower your arms, over your head towards the ground. To focus, you may want to try closing your eyes first.

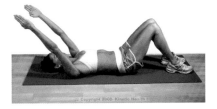

   ■ Take at least 30 seconds to slowly lower your arms to the ground.

   ■ Ensure your scapulae maintains contact with the floor for the entire motion. Stop the motion when your scapulae start to lift off the ground or when you start to use your upper trapezius muscles.

4. Check your range of motion.

5. Repeat this exercise 5 to 8 times, taking at least 30 seconds for each repetition. Your range of motion should increase slightly with each repetition.

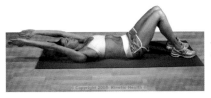

Tip: Try pretending that you are an air traffic controller, lying on the ground of the airport, and directing an aeroplane in!

Ball Circles Against the Wall - This exercise works on balance, proprioception, and coordination of the shoulder and its surrounding muscles as it moves through various ranges of motion.

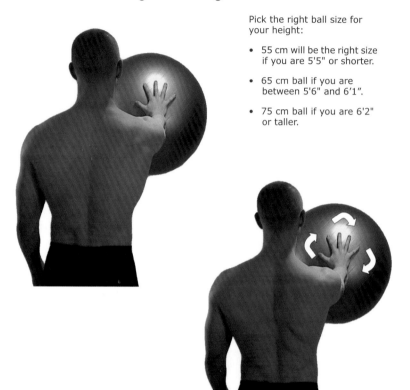

Pick the right ball size for your height:

- 55 cm will be the right size if you are 5'5" or shorter.

- 65 cm ball if you are between 5'6" and 6'1".

- 75 cm ball if you are 6'2" or taller.

1. Place the ball against the wall – at about face height – and hold it there with one hand.

2. Set your scapulae to its *normal* position, using the method described in *Setting and Activating the Scapulae - page 142*.

3. Roll 10 to 15 small clockwise circles with the ball against the wall – while keeping the scapulae set. Then repeat in an anti-clockwise direction.
   - ■ Avoid shrugging.
   - ■ Make sure you *do not* activate or use the upper trapezius muscle (from the base of your neck to your upper shoulder).
   - ■ Keep your scapulae activated throughout the exercise.

4. Repeat this exercise two to three times, for both arms.

Four Cardinal Points with the Ball - This exercise works on proprioception, balance, and coordination for your shoulder and its surrounding muscles as it moves through various ranges of motion.

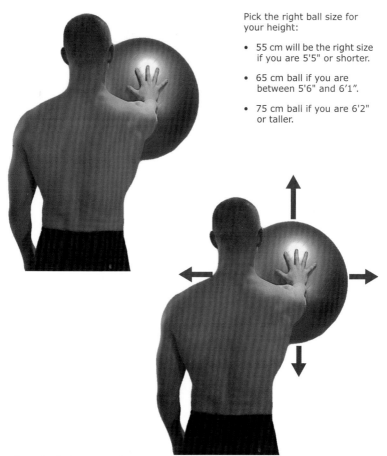

Pick the right ball size for your height:

- 55 cm will be the right size if you are 5'5" or shorter.
- 65 cm ball if you are between 5'6" and 6'1".
- 75 cm ball if you are 6'2" or taller.

1. Place the ball against the wall – at about face height – and hold it there with one hand.

2. Set your scapulae to its *normal* position, using the method described in *Setting and Activating the Scapulae - page 142.*

3. Starting from the centre, move the ball to each of the compass cardinal points, returning to the centre point after touching each compass point.

   - Make sure you *do not* activate or use the upper trapezius muscle.
   - Avoid shrugging your shoulder.

Shoulder Stretches

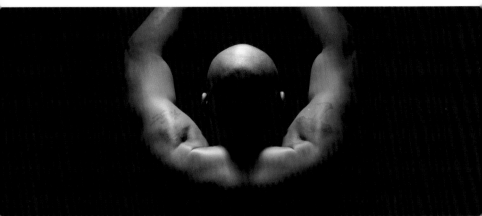

Perform the following static shoulder stretches to loosen and relax the muscles and tissues of your shoulder. Static stretching helps you to tone down your nervous system and assists in storing more energy for release when you need it. This type of stretching is great for decreasing muscle tightness.

Note: If you are involved in sporting events, then these stretches should be done **after** your have finished your sporting event. If you perform static stretching before an athletic event, you will decrease the reaction times in your nervous system. This will have the effect of reducing your performance. These are very valuable exercises, but they should be done at the right time.

Triceps and Shoulder Stretch - This is an excellent exercise that works a number of muscles including the triceps, subscapularis, serratus anterior, infraspinatus, teres minor, and teres major. You will need a long rubber tubing to do this exercise.

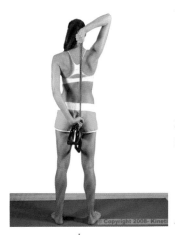

1. Stretch the tubing behind your back, holding both ends firmly.
   - The bottom hand should be positioned at the small of your back.
   - The top hand should be behind the head.
2. Keep the bottom hand relaxed.
3. With the upper hand, slowly pull the tubing upward as far as you can comfortably stretch.
   - Take at least 15 seconds to reach this maximum upwards stretch.
4. Now relax the *upper hand* back to its original position.
5. With the lower hand, slowly pull the tubing downwards as far as you can comfortably stretch.
   - Take at least 15 seconds to reach this downward maximum stretch.
   - Do not allow the upper hand to rest at your neck.
6. Repeat 3 to 5 times for BOTH sides of your body.

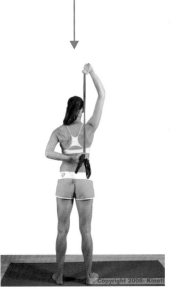

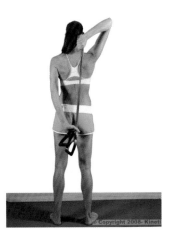

Leaning Into the Wall - This exercise stretches the subscapular and axillary muscles. The subscapularis muscle is often tight and restricted when you suffer from a shoulder injury. This muscle is used for weight lifting, racquet sports, overhead throws, pitching baseballs, playing volleyball, and in the front crawl when swimming. When this muscle is injured, you may find it difficult to sleep on your side, or find that you are unable to raise your arm up to the side.

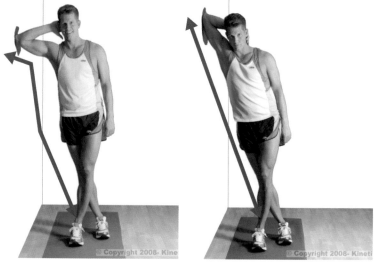

A   B

1.   Attain your starting posture:

- Place your feet about 2 feet from the wall.
- Cross your left leg over your right, as shown in Image **A**.
- Lean your elbow against the wall.
- At this point, your body should be relaxed with no tension or strain.

2.   **Exhale** as you lean into the wall, sliding your elbow up as you do so.

- Increase the stretch by leaning your upper body **into** the wall.
- Your body should form a straight line from elbow to ankle as shown in Image **B**.

3.   Hold this stretch for 15 to 30 seconds, and repeat 2 to 3 times.

4.   Repeat this exercise for the other side.

Note: Chronic restrictions in the subscapularis muscle often need to be broken up, using soft tissue techniques such as Active Release Techniques.

Foam Roller for Your Shoulders - If your shoulder muscles are really tight, you will be amazed at how quickly they relax with the following foam roller exercise. This exercise releases tightness in the posterior and lateral shoulder muscles (serratus anterior, posterior capsule, lateral/rear deltoids), in the lateral chest muscles (latissimus dorsi, teres major), and the upper back muscles (rhomboids, middle trapezius, thoracic spine).

Caution: **Never** use the foam roller along the **front** or **side** of your neck. Several critical arteries and veins (including the carotid artery) pump blood from your heart to your head and back to the heart. Crushing these with a foam roller could result in serious injury.

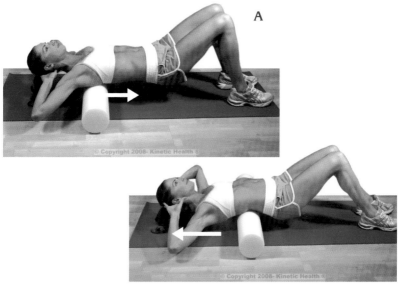

1.   Lie on your back so
     that the foam roller is perpendicular to your spine, and placed just under your shoulder.

     ■   Bend your knees and place your feet flat on the ground.
     ■   Brace your core, and lift your hips off the ground so that your body forms a straight line as shown in image **A**.

2.   Roll back and forth on the foam roller, from the top of your shoulders to your mid-back, as shown in image **B**.
     DO NOT roll onto the sides or front of your neck since you could crush delicate veins and arteries.

3.   Perform this action for 45 to 60 seconds. You may feel a little tenderness the next day, but this will quickly pass, and is a good indicator that you have released restrictions in that area.

Arm-Across-Body Stretch - This popular stretch works both the
rotator cuff and joint capsules. You should feel the stretch across the back
of your shoulder, and in the front of your shoulder and chest.

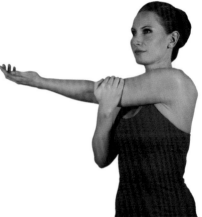

1. Stand or sit straight. Take your left arm and place it straight across your body.

2. Now take your right hand, grasp the left arm at the elbow, without torquing or twisting your body. You should feel the stretch across your shoulder, and deep within the shoulder joint

3. Hold this position for 20 to 30 seconds.

4. Repeat this exercise three to five times for each side.

Ball Stretch for the Pectoralis - This exercise targets the chest
muscles (pectoralis). Use this stretch to correcting the Anterior Posture
that is so prevalent in our culture. It opens your chest and returns your
shoulders to a neutral position.

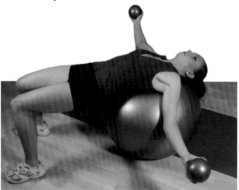

1. Lie back on an exercise ball, with your neck and shoulders resting on the ball, stomach braced, and your thighs parallel to the floor, with a 3 to 5 lb weight in each hand.

2. Extend your arms out so that they drape out over the ball.
   - ■ Relax as you do this exercise, keeping the elbows slightly bent.
   - ■ You should feel the stretch throughout your shoulders and chest.

3. Hold this position for 20 to 60 seconds. Repeat this exercise three to five times.

Tennis Ball – Posterior Shoulder Release - The back of the
shoulder often become tense and tight for many people who work at a desk or computer in a stationary position. Use a tennis ball to release tension and adhesions from specific areas along the back of your shoulder.

1. Lie on your back, on a carpet or exercise mat, with the tennis ball under the restricted area. Move or rotate your shoulder slightly to cause the tennis ball to penetrate deeper into the tissue.

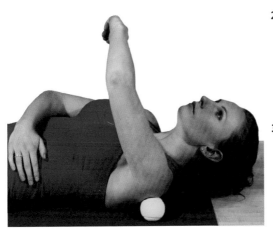

2. Once you find the point of restriction, keep working the ball at that location for an additional 15 to 30 seconds until the tension subsides.

3. Repeat for each part of your shoulder that feels tight and restricted.

Tennis Ball – Anterior Shoulder Release - Use a tennis ball to
release tension and adhesions from specific areas along the front of your shoulder.

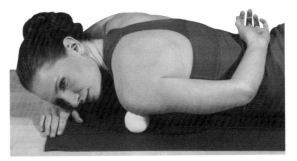

1. Lie face-down on a carpet or exercise mat. Place the tennis ball under the front of your shoulder, and gently push your weight onto it.

2. Move or rotate your body slightly to cause the tennis ball to penetrate deeper into the tissue. Once you find the point of restriction, keep the ball at that location for an additional 15 to 30 seconds until the tension subsides

3. Repeat for each part of the shoulder that feels tight and restricted.

Internal-External Shoulder Stretch - The rotator cuff, scapulae, and joint capsules of the shoulder often become tight with repeated throwing motions, racquet sports, or tasks that require you to continually reach overhead. This stretch will help to release those structures. You will need a small hand weight to perform this stretch.

A

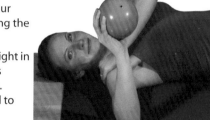

1. Lay on the floor with your shoulder blades touching the floor.
   - Hold the hand weight in your right hand as shown in image A.
   - Use your left hand to press your right shoulder into the floor.

2. Internally rotate your shoulder to bring the right hand towards the floor. See image B.
   Keep your right shoulder pinned to the ground, and do not allow your right hand to touch the floor. Hold this position of maximum stretch for 10 to 20 seconds.

B

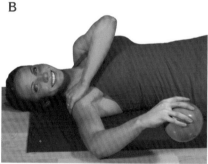

3. Rotate back to the top, and *externally* rotate your shoulder back to bring the ball beside your head.
   Don't worry if your hand does not touch the floor. Hold this position of maximum stretch for 10 to 20 seconds.

C

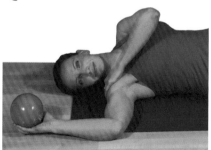

4. Repeat this action, moving between internal and external rotation, 3 to 5 times.

5. Repeat this stretch for the opposite side.

Strengthening the Shoulder

Once you have built a good awareness of your shoulder muscles, and have performed the stretching exercises, you are ready to begin strengthening the supporting muscles and tissues of your shoulder.

Beginner

Intermediate

Advanced

Attention: In many exercises, you will be asked to perform an equal number of repetitions for both sides. The goal is to create equality and stability between the muscle groups on both sides of your body.

Shoulder Shrugs with Weights - Shoulder shrugs with resistance
provided by weights act to strengthen your trapezius muscle (which runs
from the base of your skull to the bottom of your scapulae). This muscle is
used in a variety of actions including shrugging, drawing the shoulder
blades toward your midline, and pulling the shoulder blades down.

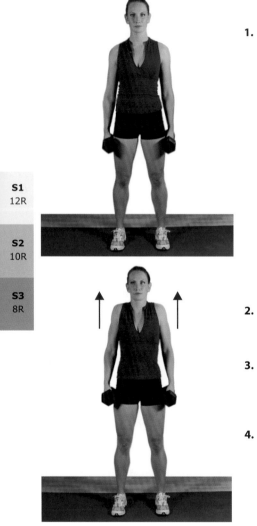

S1
12R

S2
10R

S3
8R

1. Getting Started:
   - Stand straight, with your ears centered over your shoulders, your spine in neutral position, and your feet shoulder-width apart.
   - Grasp hand weights in both hands, picking a weight that allows you to complete all three sets comfortably.
   - Ensure that your elbows are straight (but not hyper-extended) and that your thumbs brush your thighs.
   - Brace your core as shown in *How to Brace your Core! - page 15*.

2. Slowly shrug your shoulder upwards as far as you can, for a count of two.

3. Hold the shrug for a count of three then **slowly** release back down to your starting position for a count of four.

4. Repeat this exercise for the recommended number of sets and repetitions.

Shoulder Rolls - This exercise increases the mobility of your rotator cuff muscles and shoulder joint.

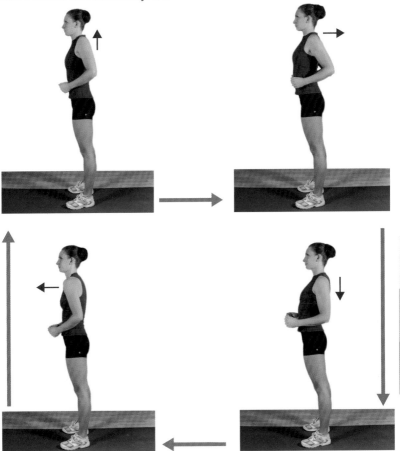

S1	10R
S2	8R
S3	6R

1. Stand or sit straight, with your ears aligned over your shoulders, and your spine in neutral position. See *Maintain Good Posture - page 77.*

2. Relax your arms and let them drop straight down.

3. Gently roll your shoulders up, back, down, and forward in a smooth rolling motion.

   ■ Hold small hand weights to increase the difficulty of this exercise.

4. Repeat this action for the required number of sets and repetitions in a *clockwise* direction, then repeat the same number of reps and sets in a *counter-clockwise* direction.

Handball Rotation - This beginner-level exercise strengthens the external rotators of the shoulder. Swimmers who use the free-style front crawl tend to be very prone to shoulder injuries due to the use of the internal rotators and the large muscles of the back and chest (latissimus dorsi and pectoralis major). But it is equally important to balance the development of these large muscle groups by strengthening the internal rotators (infraspinatus and teres minor).

Note: Much of the benefit of this exercise is derived from the use of a special soft weight (handball) of about 3 to 5 lb. The firm grip required to hold this weight causes activation of muscle groups from the shoulder all the way to the fingers, activating more areas than a traditional dumbbell weight, and also provides excellent balance-and-stabilization training.

S1
12R

S2
10R

S3
8R

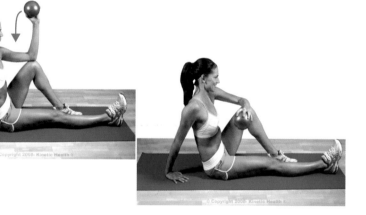

1. Sit on the floor, with the strong hand resting on the ground, and the opposite knee bent.

2. Pick up the weight with your affected arm and prop this arm on the raised knee. Your arm should be bent at the elbow to 90 degrees, pointing up to the ceiling.

3. Keep your arm at 90 degrees and slowly lower it for a count of 3 until the forearm is parallel to the ground.

4. Rotate back to the starting position – without pausing – for a count of 2.

5. Repeat this exercise for the recommended number of repetitions and sets. If the weight is correct, you should be able to execute at least 12 repetitions of these exercises, and feel fatigue after the third set.

6. Repeat this exercise for your strong side – for **exactly the same number of repetitions** as the weak side. Do not exceed this number since the goal is to balance the two sides of your body.

7. Perform 1 to 3 sets for each side.

Beginner's Push-ups - Push-ups are a great core exercise that help to improve total body fitness. Push-ups train the chest (pectoralis minor and major), triceps, and the anterior deltoids, while simultaneously stretching the biceps and back muscles. They are also very good for improving core stability.

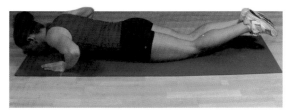

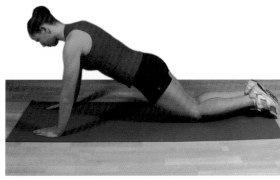

S1
8R

S2
6R

S3
4R

1. Lie face-down, palms flat on the ground with fingers facing forward, slightly more than shoulder-width apart, and supporting your body weight.
    - Bend your knees.
    - Brace your core as shown in *How to Brace your Core! - page 15.*

2. Exhale, straighten your arms, and push *up* off the floor for a count of two.
    - Keep your palms fixed at the same position.
    - Keep your knees on the ground.
    - Do not bend or arch your neck or back.
    - Push up until your arms are straight, but not hyper-extended.

3. Lower yourself for a count of 3 to return to your starting position.

4. Repeat this exercise for the recommended number of sets and repetitions.

Tip: Once you can comfortably perform 30 beginner's push-ups, you may want to advance to the Intermediate Push-ups shown on page 158.

Intermediate Push-ups - This intermediate level push-up is used to increase arm, upper body, and shoulder strength. You should feel its effects in your chest (pectorals), back of your arms (triceps), shoulders (deltoids), and rotator cuff muscles.

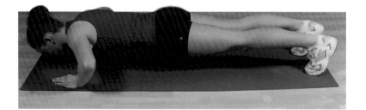

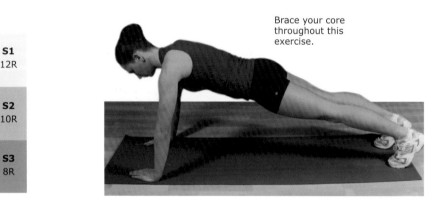

Brace your core throughout this exercise.

S1
12R

S2
10R

S3
8R

1. Lie chest-down, palms flat on the ground by your shoulders, and just a little more than shoulder-width apart. Take a deep breath, and place your feet on the floor in preparation for a plank position.

2. Exhale, straighten your arms, and push *up* off the floor.
   - Keep your palms fixed at the same position.
   - Do not bend or arch your back.

3. Hold the pushed-up position for a count of 2, then lower your chest to the floor until your arms are bent to a 90-degree angle.

4. Rest for a count of 1, and repeat from Step 2 for the recommended number of repetitions and sets.

Note: Once these become too easy, you can prop your feet up on a stability ball or bench, or raise one leg off the ground to make the push-ups harder and more challenging.

Beginner's Front Bridge - The front bridge is a classic exercise for stabilizing the shoulder and strengthening the muscles of your core. Make sure that you perform this exercise within your pain-free zone.

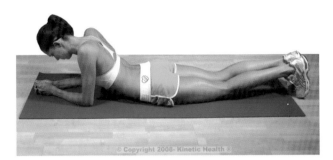

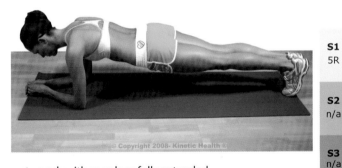

S1	5R
S2	n/a
S3	n/a

1. Lie flat on your stomach with your legs fully extended.
   - ■ Place your elbows shoulder-width apart, hands clasped together.
   - ■ Brace your core and inhale.

2. Lift your body up off the ground so that only your elbows and toes are supporting the weight of your body.
   - ■ Your body should form a straight line, from your head to your toes.
   - ■ Do not allow your spine to curve down or up.
   - ■ Do not sag, and always continue to brace your core.
   - ■ Keep your shoulders relaxed and do not hunch.
   - ■ Lengthen your body through your spine as you exhale.

3. Hold the bridge for 10 seconds, then slowly lower yourself back to the ground.

4. Perform this exercise 5 times in total.

Beginner's Side Bridge – Knee Bent - This very effective
exercise targets your shoulders and core abdominal muscles. Use this
exercise to strengthen your core and to power all the actions of your body.

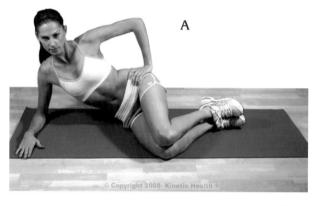

A

S1
3R

S2
n/a

S3
n/a

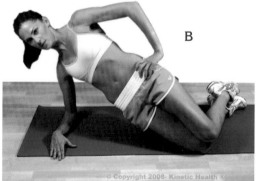

B

1. Lie on your side as shown in image **A** and brace your core.

2. Lift your body up off the ground so that only your arm and knees are
    supporting the weight of your body as shown in image **B**.
    - Your body should form a straight line, from your head to your knees.
    - Do not allow your spine to curve forward or back.
    - Do not sag, and always continue to brace your core.

3. Hold the side-bridge for 10 to 15 seconds, breathing normally, then slowly
    lower yourself back to the ground. It is important to *initially* hold this
    bridge position for just 10 seconds to prevent injuries, build your
    endurance, and develop the right type of muscle tissue (slow twitch
    muscles).

4. Wait 10 to 15 seconds before repeating this exercise for a total of three
    times on this side.

Lasso with a Handball - This intermediate-level exercise improves coordination, range of motion, and strength. It acts to strengthen the deltoids, triceps, upper trapezius, and rotator cuff muscles.

Note: Much of the benefit of this exercise is derived from the special soft weight (handballs weighing about 3 to 5 lb). The firm grip required to hold this ball causes activation of more muscle groups than a traditional hand weight, and is excellent for balance and stabilization training.

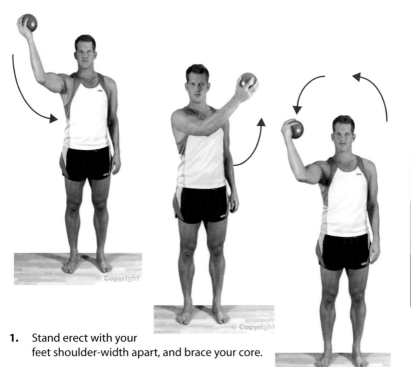

S1	10R
S2	8R
S3	6R

1. Stand erect with your feet shoulder-width apart, and brace your core.

2. Clasp the handball with a **firm** grip.

3. With your arm extended but elbows slightly bent, make large circular motions, as if you are drawing a large lasso.

4. Repeat this motion for the recommended number of repetitions and sets in a clockwise direction, then reverse the direction, and repeat for the same number of times in a counter-clockwise direction.

5. Perform exactly the **same number** of repetitions and motions with the other hand.

Note: In all these exercises, it is important to exercise both sides of the body (injured and non-injured) equally.

Lateral Raise with Tubing - This intermediate-level exercise
activates your core and strengthens the serratus anterior and latissimus
dorsi muscles. The serratus anterior muscle is responsible for the
protraction of the scapulae, such as when you throw a punch. The
latissimus dorsi is a large back muscle, which helps to pull your upper
arms down and in front of your body, as well as letting you rotate your
upper arm inward.

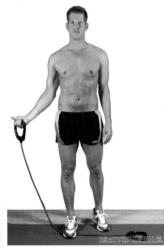

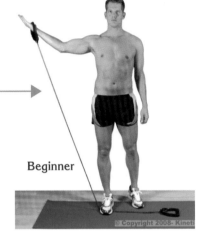

Beginner

S1
10R

S2
8R

S3
6R

1. Stand on the tubing so that it is
    securely under your foot, and cannot
    escape to hit you on the head.

2. Hold the handle with your right
    hand, palm facing outwards, thumb
    up.

3. Brace your core and raise your arm
    straight up the side of your body for
    a count of 2.

    ■ Keep your arm partially bent.
    ■ Only raise the tubing to a
       height that remains pain-free.
       Do not exceed this distance.

4. Slowly return to the starting position
    for a count of 3.

5. Repeat this exercise, on both sides,
    for the recommended number of
    repetitions and sets.

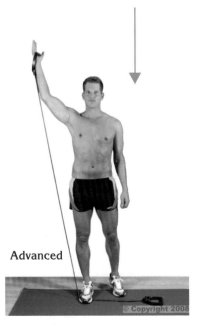

Advanced

Work those Triceps and Shoulders - Use this exercise to
strengthen your triceps and shoulders, and to counter-balance the power of
your biceps.

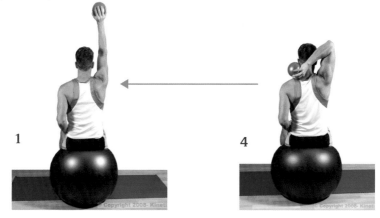

1

4

1. Sit balanced on the ball, feet planted firmly on the ground,
   your spine in neutral position, with the handball grasped
   firmly in your raised right hand.

2. Exhale and lower the right behind your *right shoulder.*

3. Raise your right hand straight up (for a count of 2), then
   exhale and lower the ball (for a count of 3) to your *opposite
   (left) shoulder.*

4. Return to the starting position, and repeat this exercise for
   the recommended number of repetitions and sets.

5. Perform this exercise for both sides of your body.

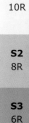

S1
10R

S2
8R

S3
6R

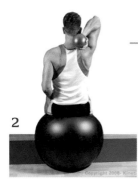

2

3

Swiss Ball Row - This exercise strengthens the upper back stabilizers such as the rhomboids (between your shoulder blades) and mid-trapezius. Use this exercise to improve your ability to retract your scapulae towards your vertebrae and to improve your core stability.

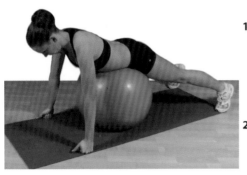

1. Lay on your stomach on the exercise ball. Brace both feet to keep your balance and to prevent yourself from sliding off the ball.

2. Slowly lift your arms up, pulling your shoulder blades towards the centre line.

S1
10R

S2
8R

S3
6R

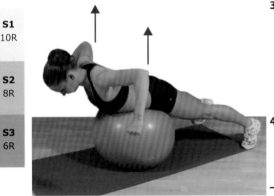

3. Now rotate your shoulders to bring your arms up and parallel to your head.

   ■ Hold for a count of 2, then slowly lower your arms.

4. Repeat this exercise for the recommended number of sets and repetitions.

Note: As you increase in strength, you can choose to perform this exercise with a weight that you can lift comfortably 10 times.

You may want to start with a 2-to-5 lb weight, and work upwards to heavier weights as your strength increases.

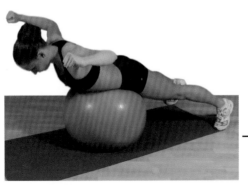

Throw a Javelin - This exercise activates your core while strengthening your rotator cuff, deltoids (which moves the arm away from the body), latissimus dorsi, and trapezius. This functional exercise is great for combining whole body movement with shoulder stabilization.

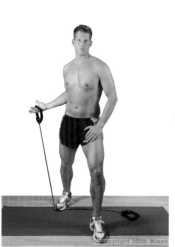

1. Start in a semi-lunge position, with the rubber tubing held securely under the back foot, and the handle in your right hand.

    ■ The tubing should feel taut at hip level.
    ■ Palm faces upwards.
    ■ Brace your core and exhale.

2. Pull your right hand up and forward, as if you are throwing a javelin.

    ■ Slightly increase your lunge posture.
    ■ Hold the extended position for a count of 2.

3. Return to the starting position and perform the exercise for the recommended number of sets and repetitions.

4. Repeat this exercise on the opposite side for the *same* number of repetitions and sets.

S1
10R

S2
8R

S3
6R

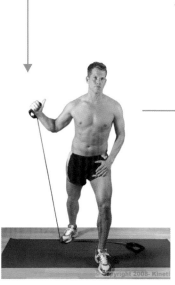

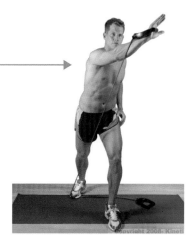

Draw a Sword - Use this exercise to strengthen your rotator cuff while activating key core stability muscles. Perform this exercise within a pain-free range of motion. If you feel pain, reduce the tension in the tubing and try again.

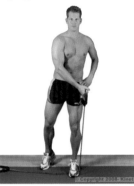

1. Stand on the tubing so that it is secure under your left foot, and cannot snap out.

   - The handle should be on the left side.
   - Reach across with your right hand and grasp the handle firmly, thumb facing out, right hand by your hip.
   - Ensure you have sufficient tension. The tubing should not be floppy.
   - Brace your core.

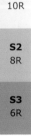

S1
10R

S2
8R

S3
6R

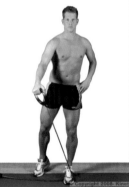

2. Pull the tubing (for a count of 2) diagonally out from your left hip, past your right hip, and up above your head as if you are drawing and brandishing a sword.

   - Hold the extended position for a count of 2.
   - Do not lock your elbows when you extend your arm, and maintain an upright posture throughout the entire action.
   - The tubing should feel tight and stretched at the top of the draw.

3. Return to the starting position and perform the recommended number of sets and repetitions, for both sides of your body.

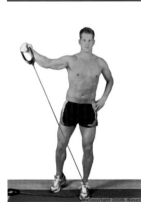

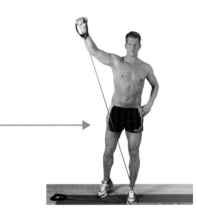

Prone Y on the Floor - This exercise focuses on the trapezius, rhomboids, rotator cuff, and paraspinal muscles of the upper back. It works to increase neuromuscular performance and acts to stabilize the scapulae, which performs a critical role in the biomechanics of your shoulder.

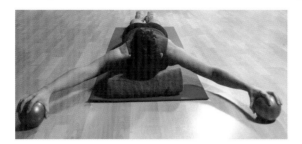

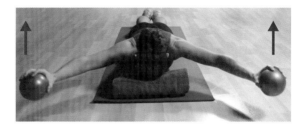

S1
10R

S2
8R

S3
6R

1. Lie face-down on a firm surface. For comfort, place a rolled-up towel under your forehead to support your head.

2. Grip a small weighted handball (1 to 5 lb) in each hand, and position your arms above your head.

3. Brace your core and exhale.

4. Raise both arms off the floor.
   - Hold for a count of 3.
   - You should feel the muscles of your scapulae working.
   - Keep a firm grip on the handballs. This gripping action helps to work the full kinetic chain from your shoulder to your arms.

5. Slowly lower your arms to the starting position.

6. Perform the recommended number of sets and repetitions.

Prone T on the Floor - This exercise focuses on strengthening the rhomboids, deltoids, trapezius, scapulae, and paraspinal muscles of the upper back. After an injury, it is essential to strengthen and re-train the scapulae since it is a key link in the shoulder and is actively involved in retraction, protraction, upward and downward rotation, as well as elevation and depression of the shoulder.

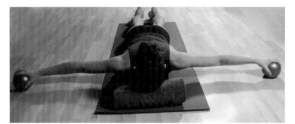

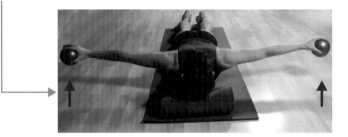

S1
10R

S2
8R

S3
6R

1. Lie face-down on a firm surface. For comfort, place a rolled-up towel under your forehead to support your head.

2. Grip a small weighted handball (1 to 5 lb) in each hand, and stretch both arms out, keeping them aligned with your shoulder.

3. Gently brace your core, and exhale.

4. Raise both arms off the floor.
   - Hold for a count of 3.
   - Maintain a slight bend in your elbow.
   - Keep your arms aligned with your shoulders.
   - Keep a firm grip on the handballs. This gripping action helps to work the full kinetic chain from your shoulder to your arms.

5. Slowly lower your arms to the starting position.

6. Perform the recommended number of repetitions and sets for this exercise.

Prone L: Retract Your Scapulae - This exercise focuses on strengthening the rhomboids, posterior deltoids, rotator cuff, scapulae, and paraspinals of the upper back. The rhomboid muscles are often overworked carrying heavy loads on your back, holding a poor posture from working on a computer, and engaging rowing and racquet sports.

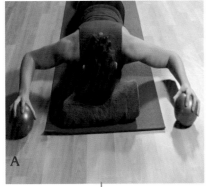

A

1. Lie face-down on a firm surface. For comfort, place a rolled up towel under your forehead to support your head.

2. Grip a small weighted handball in each hand, and stretch both arms out as shown in image A, with the elbows bent to a 90-degree angle.

3. Brace your core and exhale.

4. Raise both arms off the floor, and try to pinch your shoulder blades together. To get the correct action, imagine that you are squeezing an orange between your shoulder blades.

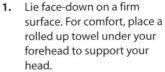

S1	S2	S3
10R	8R	6R

- ■ Hold for a count of 3.
- ■ Keep your arms aligned with your shoulders.
- ■ Keep a firm grip on the handballs. This gripping action helps to work the full kinetic chain from your shoulder through to your arms.

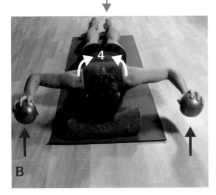

B

5. Lower your arms to the starting position.

6. Perform the recommended number of repetitions and sets for this exercise.

Stabilize and Strengthen Your Scapulae - This exercise
focuses on strengthening and stabilizing the muscles of the scapulae. A
stable and strong scapula is essential for good shoulder joint function.
Scapular motion affects rotator cuff stability, neck and mid-back function,
and the function of the muscles on the front of your chest.

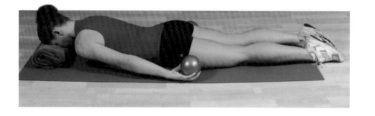

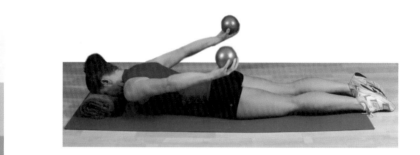

S1
10R

S2
8R

S3
6R

1. Lie face-down on a firm surface. For comfort, place a rolled-up towel
   under your forehead to support your head.

2. Grip a small weighted handball (1 to 5 lb) in each hand, and stretch both
   arms down the length of your body.

3. Brace your core and exhale.

4. Raise both arms off the floor.
   - Hold for a count of three.
   - Keep your arms straight, slightly bent at the elbows.
   - Keep a firm grip on the handballs. This gripping action helps to
     work the full kinetic chain from your shoulder through
     to your arms.

5. Lower your arms to the starting position and repeat from step 3.

6. Perform the recommended number of repetitions and sets.

Performance Care for the Shoulder

Only use the remainder of these shoulder exercises if you are able to comfortably and easily perform the exercises in *Advanced Shoulder Workout - page 93*, and remain completely injury-free. These are advanced shoulder exercises that integrate and use multiple elements of your shoulder's kinetic chain.

Benefits of Exercise Tubing

Exercise tubing is an ideal tool for building strength as it accommodates easily to all levels of strength and allows you to easily increase resistance by shortening the tubing. Tubing exercises performed in a standing position force you to activate and stabilize your core as you perform the complete range of motion. For all tubing exercises, be sure to:

■ Anchor the tubing securely to either a closed door or other stable, non-moving object. Make sure no one can open the door while you exercise.

■ Increase or decrease resistance by either shortening or lengthening the tubing, or by increasing or decreasing the diameter of the tubing.

■ Perform all actions smoothly, with no sudden jerking motions.

Standing Row with Tubing -

By using the exercise tubing in an upright position you will be working your entire kinetic chain, from your core through the rotator cuff, chest, arms, core, hips, and legs.

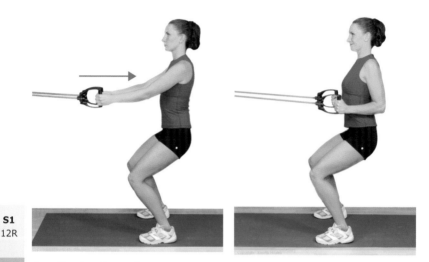

S1
12R

S2
10R

S3
8R

1. **Getting Started:**
   - Anchor your exercise tubing securely to a closed door (or other anchor) at a low level.
   - Hold the tubing with both hands, position yourself to get sufficient and equal tension in the tubing, and get into a squat position. The lower the squat position, the harder the exercise is to do.

2. Brace your core muscles, and hold them in this braced position throughout the exercise, while continuing to breathe normally.

3. Bend your arms, and pull your arms back towards your torso for a count of 2.
   - Keep your arms snug against your body as you do this.
   - Do not arch or curve your back.
   - Keep your core braced.

4. Hold this position for a count of 1, and then release slowly for a count of 3 to return to your starting position, staying upright throughout the release.

5. Repeat this exercise for the recommended numbers of sets and repetitions.

Strengthening the Latissimus Dorsi - You will often see people doing this exercise in the gym with a cable machine. But you can also do it at home with exercise tubing and a closed door! This exercise really works your latissimus dorsi, rhomboids, and shoulder muscles.

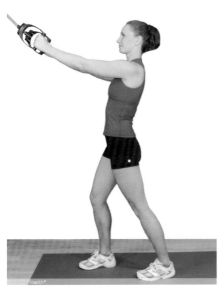

1. **Getting Started**:

   ■ Anchor your exercise tubing securely and safely to a closed door, at shoulder height.

   ■ Stand facing the door, feet shoulder-width apart.

   ■ Extend your arms in front of you and pull the exercise tubing tight at about shoulder height. If necessary adjust your location to ensure tautness of the exercise tubing.

   ■ Brace your core muscles (*How to Brace your Core! - page 15*).

2. Exhale, and in a slow, smooth motion pull the exercise tubing towards your chest for a count of 2, until your hands are almost touching your chest.

3. Hold this position for a count of 1, then slowly release for a count of 3 to return to your starting position. Keep your back straight and aligned, and do not lean forward during the return.

4. Repeat this exercise for the recommended number of sets and repetitions.

S1
12R

S2
10R

S3
8R

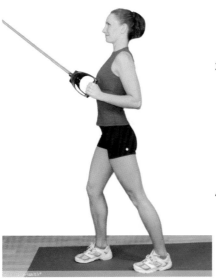

Chest Fly with Tubing - Shoulder and neck injuries typically affect the function and strength of your chest and shoulders. This exercise uses exercise tubing to improve your shoulder retraction and protraction, and increases shoulder mobility and strength in the chest muscles.

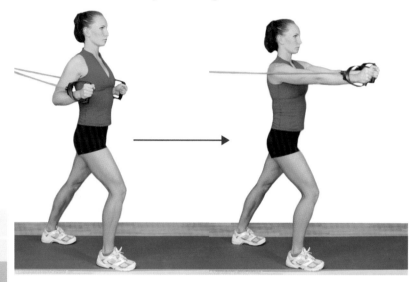

S1
12R

S2
10R

S3
8R

1. **Getting Started**:
   - Anchor your exercise tubing securely and safely to a closed door, at shoulder height.
   - Stand with your back to the door, feet shoulder-width apart, with one foot about 8 inches ahead of the other, and your body in a lunge position.
   - Grasp the ends of the exercise tubing and bring the tubing to chest height beside your body. Keep your thumbs up, and elbows and shoulders aligned as you maintain tension in the tubing.
   - Brace your core muscles (*How to Brace your Core! - page 15*) throughout the exercise, but continue breathing normally.

2. In a slow, smooth motion push the exercise tubing forward for a count of 2 until your palms face each other and your arms are almost straight.

3. Hold this position for a count of 1, and then release **SLOWLY** for a count of 3 to return to your starting position. Keep your back straight and aligned, and do not lean forward during the return.

4. Repeat this exercise for the recommended number of sets and repetitions.

Chest Pull-Over with Tubing - This great little exercise can be easily performed with a closed door and exercise tubing. It works the muscles of your chest, shoulders, back, and core!

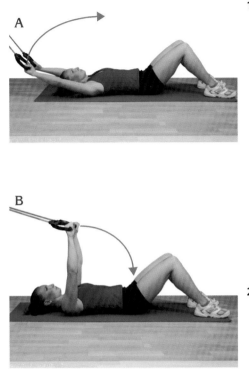

A

B

C

1. **Getting Started**:
   - ▪ Anchor your exercise tubing securely to a closed door, at a low level.
   - ▪ Lie on the floor with your head towards the door.
   - ▪ Position your body as shown in image **A** and ensure you have sufficient tension when your arms are stretched over your head.
   - ▪ Brace your core muscles (*How to Brace your Core! - page 15*).

2. Exhale, keep your arm slightly bent, and pull the tubing down to your hips for a count of 2 in a smooth, continuous motion.

3. Hold this position for a count of 1, and then release **SLOWLY** for a count of 3 to return to your starting position.

4. Repeat this exercise for the recommended numbers of sets and repetitions.

Note: Breathe normally throughout this exercise. *Do not* hold your breath.

S1	12R
S2	10R
S3	8R

Beginner's Four-Point Kneeling - This is not only a great core exercise, but it is also an excellent exercise for grooving your neuro-motor system. Four-point kneeling teaches your body to transfer energy from your lower extremity through your core to the upper extremity. Best of all, it acts to increase the stability and neuromuscular control of your whole body!

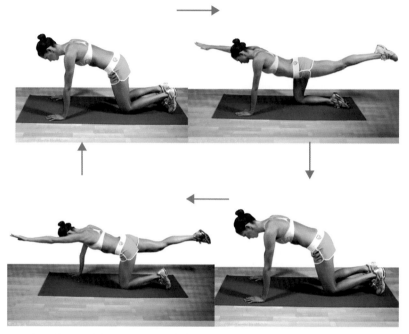

S1
10R

S2
8R

S3
6R

1. **Starting position**: Kneel on all fours.
   - Keep your hands and knees planted firmly on the ground as you face forward.
   - Keep your spine in neutral position.
   - Inhale and brace your core.
2. Exhale and slowly straighten your **right arm** and **left leg**.
   - Keep your arm and leg parallel to the floor, and aligned with your torso.
   - Maintain your spine in neutral position and avoid tilting your back or pelvis.
3. Hold this position for 10 seconds.
4. Slowly lower your arm and leg to the starting position.
5. Perform the entire sequence for the recommended number of sets and repetitions.
6. Repeat the above steps with the **left arm and right leg**.

Advanced Four-Point Kneeling - This advanced version of Four-Point Kneeling increases both shoulder and core stability, allowing you to direct more power from your core to your extremities. This exercise increases neuromuscular control and improves the strength of the abdominals, erector spinae, gluteals and hamstring muscles.

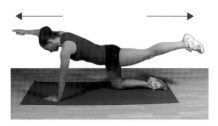

1. **Starting position**: Kneel on all fours as in *Beginner's Four-Point Kneeling - page 176*.

2. Exhale and slowly straighten the **right arm** and **left leg** as described in *Beginner's Four-Point Kneeling - page 176*.
   - ■ Hold for a count of 3.

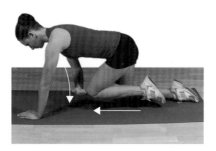

3. Now curve the extended arm under and across your body, while tucking in the extended knee to touch the curved arm. Don't touch the floor. Hold this position for 2 seconds.

4. Now stretch the right arm out so that it is perpendicular to the body, and extend the **left** leg.
   - ■ Hold this position for a count of 3.

5. Slowly return your arm and leg to the starting position.

6. Perform the entire sequence for the recommended number of sets and repetitions.

7. Repeat the above steps with the **left arm** and **right leg**.

S1
12R

S2
10R

S3
8R

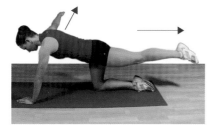

Medicine Ball Wood Chop

- This dynamic exercise simulates the action involved in chopping wood. It develops core strength, improves speed and reaction time, and increases your neuromuscular control. This is a great exercise for improving your golf swing.

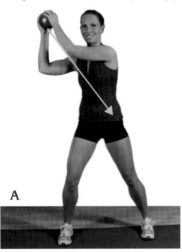

A

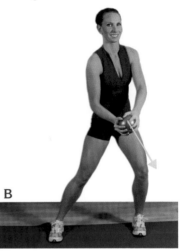

B

S1
12R

S2
10R

S3
8R

1. Hold a moderate weight exercise or medicine ball in both hands.

2. Raise both hands to one side of your body as shown in image **A**.

3. Transfer your weight and bring the ball diagonally down towards the opposite knee.

4. Perform the entire sequence for the recommended number of sets and repetitions.

5. Repeat the same number of sets and repetitions for the other side of your body.

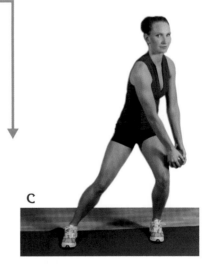

C

Alternating Dumbbell Press on Ball - This is basically a dumbbell bench press, but by performing it on a ball with alternating hands, you are able to activate and use more of your core and upper and lower extremities, and increase your neuromuscular control.

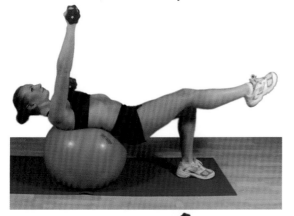

S1
12R

S2
10R

S3
8R

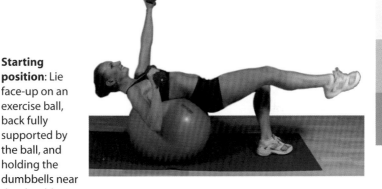

1. **Starting position**: Lie face-up on an exercise ball, back fully supported by the ball, and holding the dumbbells near the shoulders.

   - Activate your scapulae and keep them activated throughout the exercise. See *Setting and Activating the Scapulae - page 142*.
   - Brace your core muscles. See (*How to Brace your Core! - page 15*.
   - Raise your right leg, while keeping your left foot firmly on the ground.

2. Raise the right dumbbell straight up above your shoulder for a count of 2, keeping your back and shoulder flexed.

3. Return the right dumbbell to the starting position for a count of 3, and repeat the procedure for the left dumbbell.

4. Switch your leg positions halfway through the set.

5. Perform the recommended number of sets and repetitions, alternating the leg positions halfway through each set.

Forward Bridge – Advanced

Forward Bridge – Advanced - This advanced forward bridge alternates movements of the hands and legs while in the Plank position. This difficult exercise should not be attempted until you have mastered the Beginner's Front Bridge. This is a very good exercise for strengthening the rectus abdominis, transversus abdominis, and internal oblique muscles, as well as the muscles along the abdominal wall which act as a counter-balance to the transversospinalis.

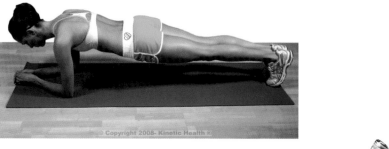

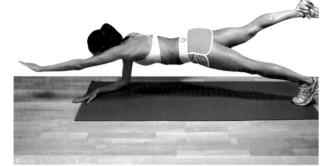

S1
6R

S2
4R

S3
2R

1. Lay flat on your stomach with your legs fully extended. Place your elbows shoulder-width apart, hands lightly clasped. Brace your core and inhale.

2. Exhale and assume the plank position detailed in *Beginner's Front Bridge - page 159*.

3. Now raise your **left arm and right leg** so that they are aligned with your body. Hold this extended position for 10 seconds.

4. Return to the starting position in Step 2.

5. Repeat the steps with the **right arm and left leg**.

6. Repeat the exercise for both sides, for the recommended number of sets and repetitions.

Front-to-Side Bridge

- Bridge exercises are excellent for strengthening your core. The Front-to-Side Bridge is an advanced exercise that combines the movement patterns of both the front and side bridge, and acts to stabilize your shoulders, core, hips, abdominal obliques, and lower extremities.

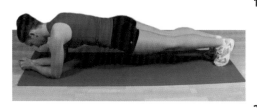

1. **Starting position**: Begin on the floor in the classic front bridge or plank position as shown in *Beginner's Front Bridge - page 159*. Brace your core and inhale.

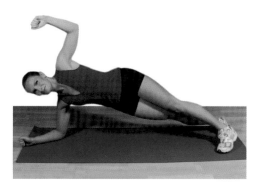

2. Turn your torso slightly so that you can lift your **left arm** into the air.

   - Slightly stagger your feet so you have a base of support while in this position.
   - Your upper body weight should be distributed along the right forearm.
   - Hold the side bridge position for 2 seconds.

S1	S2	S3
12R	10R	8R

3. Return to the starting front bridge position.

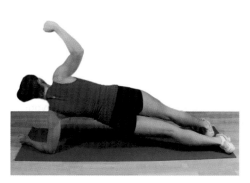

4. Repeat from step 1 for the opposite side, lifting your **right arm** up as you turn your torso and distribute your body weight onto the left side.

5. Repeat this sequence for the recommended number of repetitions and sets.

Russian Twist with Medicine Ball -

This advanced exercise really works and strengthens the rectus abdominis, external and internal oblique abdominal muscles, and the transversus abdominis. These muscles are involved in twisting motions such as those in golf and baseball. The exercise and medicine balls add elements of balance and proprioception to your actions.

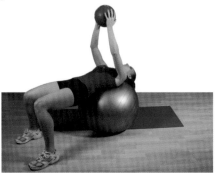

S1
12R

S2
10R

S3
8R

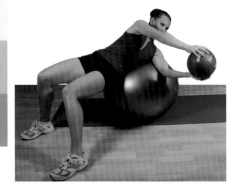

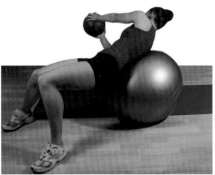

1. Starting Position:
   - Sit on a medium-size exercise ball and hold a weighted medicine ball close to your chest with both hands.
   - Roll forward so that your back is resting comfortably on the exercise ball.
   - Keep your knees perpendicular to the ground, and your ankles and knees aligned.
   - Activate your gluteal muscles and keep the contraction throughout the exercise.
   - Keeping a slight bend at the elbows, lift the medicine ball straight up, above your chin.

2. Brace your core, inhale, and twist your torso to the right for a count of 2.

3. Hold this position for 2 seconds

4. Exhale as you return to starting position for a count of 2.

5. Repeat from Step 2 for the opposite side.

6. Perform the recommended number of repetitions and sets for both sides of your body.

Push-ups with Unequal Hands - So, you have done all those other push-ups, and are finding them just a little too easy, and perhaps boring. Try this challenging version to really strengthen those muscles in your core and upper extremity. Do not perform this push-up until you are able to easily complete the exercises in the *Advanced Shoulder* routine.

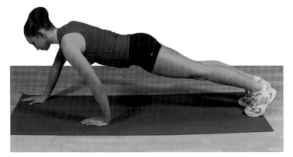

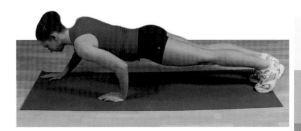

S1
10R

S2
8R

S3
6R

1. **Getting Started**:
   - Get into a standard push-up position.
   - Place your right hand parallel to your face.
   - Place your left hand beside your waist.
   - Play around with these hand positions to increase or decrease the level of difficulty.
   - Exhale, straighten your arms, and push *up* off the floor for a count of 2.

2. Brace your core. See *How to Brace your Core! - page 15.*

3. Hold the pushed-up position for a count of 2, then lower yourself slowly to the ground for a count of 3.

4. Immediately rest for a count of 1, and repeat from Step 2.

5. Repeat this exercise for the recommended number of sets and repetitions.

6. Then switch your arm positions and repeat for the opposite side, for the same number of repetitions and sets.

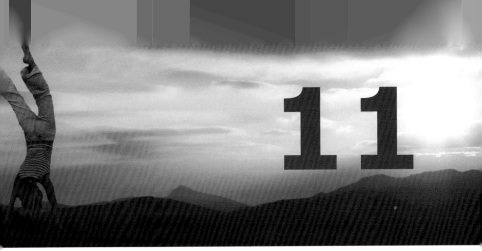

Self Care Tips and Hints

Since soft-tissue and joint injuries are very common, it is good to know what you can do to take care of yourself when it happens. Rapid treatment is essential for ensuring quick recovery from these injuries.

The tips and hints we are providing in this chapter relate to the care of sprain/strain or minor joint injuries that occur due to repetitive actions, trauma, poor body mechanics, inflammation, excessive stress to the muscles and tissues of your body, and muscle imbalances within your kinetic chain. They do not apply to serious trauma or emergency situations.

Note: In this book, we are **not** talking about dealing with traumatic injuries involving open wounds, bleeding, impaled objects, extreme force injuries, etc. For such cases, seek immediate care from your medical practitioner.

For most non-traumatic soft tissue injuries, start self-care with the following:

- Cold Therapy ....see page 186.
- Heat Therapy ....see page 188.
- Epsom Salt Baths ....see page 190.
- Benefits of Rest ....see page 191.
- Exercise ....see page 192.

Cold Therapy

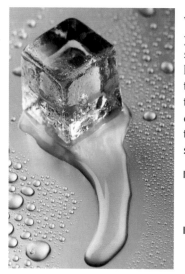

When you have a soft-tissue injury, you will often feel pain and muscle spasms. Your area of injury may become inflamed and swollen due to the tearing of blood vessels and the release of fluids into the damaged area. Your first goal in treating most soft-tissue injuries should be to:

- Slow the release of hormones and chemicals that cause the pain and inflammation.

- Reduce inflammation by decreasing the movement of fluids into the area.

The easiest and most effective means to do this is **Cold Therapy.** Cold therapy helps numb the nerves, reduce pain signals being sent to the brain, reduce muscle spasms, reduce swelling by constricting the blood vessels, reduce cell death by decreasing the rate of metabolism, and reduce blood flow to the area.

Cold therapy should be the FIRST treatment for inflammation! And...it should be applied within the first 48 hours of injury–the sooner, the better. In many cases, applying ice within the first hour can reduce healing times by as much as 50%.

Yes, we know that HEAT sounds much more tempting and comforting – especially when you are in pain or are living in colder climates. But, remember that heat therapy increases blood flow to an area, and therefore can cause more inflammation and pain... something you want to avoid during the acute stages of inflammation!

Tips and Hints for Icing

■ While icing, elevate the injured area – preferably above the heart – to reduce swelling by moving blood away from the affected area.

■ Ice every two to three hours, but first make sure that the area being iced has warmed up and is no longer numb.

■ Prevent frostbite by not allowing the ice pack to sit directly on your skin. Use a thin towel in-between.

When Not to Ice!

Do not use Cold Therapy if the person:

■ Is unconscious, unable to communicate, or has no sensation in the injured area.

■ Tends to develop a rash or blisters when exposed to cold.

■ Has circulatory problems.

■ Has Raynaud's disease, rheumatoid or gouty arthritis, kidney malfunctions, or hyperthyroidism.

Icing with an Ice-Pack

• Place a thin cloth on the injured area.

• Apply the ice-pack to the injured area.

• Keep the ice-pack against the affected area until it feels numb.

You should first feel **cold**, then a **burning sensation**, followed by **aching**, then **numbness**. If you don't feel numb, then you haven't iced for long enough.

• This process takes about 15 to 20 minutes. Never longer!

• Do NOT allow the skin to freeze...you are not trying to get frost-bite.

• Leave a minimum of one hour between each icing session to allow your tissues to warm up.

Ice Massage

Ice massage can be more effective than regular icing.

• Fill small paper cups with water and keep them in your freezer till frozen.

• Peel the top of the cup back to expose the ice.

• Massage the ice over the injured area in small circular motions, allowing the ice to melt away.

• Use a towel to catch the melting water.

• To **prevent tissue damage**, only perform ice massage for a maximum of 7 to 9 minutes.

Heat Therapy

Without a doubt, Heat Therapy feels much nicer and more comforting than Cold Therapy. But problems can arise when heat therapy is used too soon after an injury or trauma. In fact, the early use of heat therapy by our patients is often the primary reason for the increased time required to resolve their soft-tissue injuries.

Heat Therapy should only be used *after inflammation has subsided.* Never use heat therapy within the first 72 hours of an acute injury. Applying heat to soft tissues (muscles, ligaments, and tendons) while the area is still inflamed and swollen will only aggravate the injured tissues. During the first 72 hours, cold therapy provides much more effective and appropriate relief.

Benefits of Heat Therapy

Once the inflammation has subsided, you can apply heat to the affected area to help restore flexibility, relieve muscle cramping, reduce arthritic symptoms, and most of all, to increase the rate of healing by increasing blood-flow to the area.

The power of heat therapy comes from its depth of penetration and its ability to increase circulatory and neurological function. Increasing circulation results in increased delivery of oxygen and nutrients to the affected area while at the same time displacing waste by-products. Heat affects the nervous system by stimulating the sensory receptors in your skin. This has the effect of decreasing the transmission of pain signals to your brain, thereby reducing muscle spasms and episodes of acute pain.

Types of Heat Therapy

The effectiveness of heat therapy varies from individual to individual. Each person needs to experiment to determine which therapy is best suited to their condition. There are two primary types of heat therapy:

■ **Moist Heat**: Moist heat therapy includes hot baths, heated whirlpools, hot packs, or hot moist towels. Many people feel they get better depth of penetration with moist heat.

■ **Dry heat**: Dry heat therapy includes dry saunas, electric heating pads, and heat lamps. These can be very effective forms of heat therapy but they also tend to dehydrate the individual, so remember to drink lots of fluids when you use dry heat therapy.

For how long should you apply heat therapy? For a minor, superficial injury you may only want to use heat therapy for 10 to 20 minutes. For chronic injuries, you may need to apply heat therapy for 20 to 35 minutes.

Heat Treatment with a Hot Towel

- Dampen an old, clean towel (towels may discolour with this process).
- Heat the moist towel in a microwave for one to two minutes. Check the temperature of the towel, and heat for another minute if necessary.
- Carefully remove the moist hot towel (don't give yourself a steam burn) and wrap the hot towel with a dry towel (to prevent burns, and to retain the heat).
- Apply the hot towel to the affected area until your muscles relax and warm up, and your skin turns slightly rosy.
- Stop after 15 to 20 minutes. Do not re-apply for at least 1 to 2 hours.

Attention: Always use caution with Heat Therapy. Use only moderate heat to avoid burning the soft tissue. Do not use heat treatment if you suffer from one or more of the following conditions: cancer, diabetes mellitus, tendency to hemorrhage, decreased sensations, peripheral vascular disease, acute inflammation, cognitive impairment, deep vein thrombosis, dermatitis, heart disease, hypertension (high blood pressure), skin lesions, or open wounds. If in doubt, consult your physician!
Try to avoid using Heat Therapy at night, or when you are in bed. You are more likely to fall asleep with the heating pad, and that could be dangerous since it can cause burns and overheating.

Epsom Salt Baths

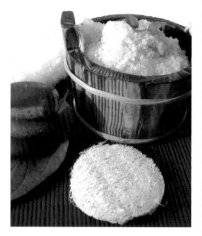

Grandmother's magic home remedy for aches and pains...epsom salts. Soaking in an epsom salt bath is one of the best things you can (and should) do for your body.

Epsom salts (magnesium sulfate) have a high concentration of magnesium, which help to draw out inflammation – pushing chemicals and toxins out of muscles and joints, relaxing muscles, and moisturizing skin.

But, remember that epsom salt baths is another form of Heat Therapy, and therefore all the rules that apply to Heat Therapy also apply to epsom salt baths.

After long runs, a hot bath with epsom salts is recommended to reduce the pain in aching legs. We recommend soaking in an epsom salt bath at least once a week to reduce daily aches and pains. You can also use epsom salts for reducing inflammation from localized soft-tissue injuries.

Using Epsom Salts Locally

- Fill a bucket of hot water, add one cup of epsom salts, and soak your sore feet or hands.
- Dip a wash cloth in epsom-salt-drenched water, and wrap it around your sore achilles tendon to reduce inflammation.
- Soak a cloth in epsom salt water, wring it out, and place it over a sore or painful area. Now wrap a tensor bandage or towel around everything to keep the heat in, and to hold the epsom-salt-soaked towel in place! It works wonders!

Make an Epsom Salt Bath:

Mix two (2) cups of epsom salts in lots of hot water.

Soak in the bath and let the Epsom Salts do their magic!

Benefits of Rest

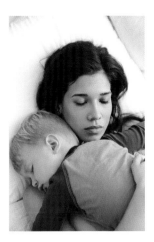

Rest, in our busy world, is becoming an increasingly rare commodity. But it is an essential component for healing your body.

Your body needs rest and sleep in order to function properly and to repair itself. While you sleep, your body performs much of its maintenance and renewal functions.

If you have any type of soft-tissue injury (caused by sports, career, home care, or just daily activities), you must *rest* that area to give it a chance to recover properly.

Lack of sleep results in decreased immune function, increased potential for disease (heart disease, stroke, cancer), decreased hormone production (human growth hormone), decreased tissue repair, decreased cognitive function, decreased fat metabolism, depression, increased inflammation, and even decreased life span.

Some very interesting research has come out of the National Academy of Science about the effects of sleep deprivation. Sleep deprivation causes an elevated level of the stress hormone, corticosterone. Increased levels of this hormone causes a reduction in the function of brain cells. This, in turn, has been directly related to problems in concentration and other possible cognitive issues. A little sad, but lack of sleep may even reduce cognitive function so much that you don't even realize there is a problem.

We have found that our patients' lack of rest and sleep is one of the primary reasons for a slow or delayed recovery from an injury. Avoid over-using an injured area before it is recovered as that can cause further injury, more inflammation, and increased healing time.

How much sleep you require will vary based on several factors, including your diet (good diet, bad diet), environmental factors (smoking, drinking), quality of sleep, genetics, and current injuries. Even the quality of light that you are exposed to will affect the amount of sleep you need (spending a long time in front of your computer disrupts your circadian rhythm). In general terms we recommend at least 7 to 8 hours of sleep per night.

Reducing sleep by as little as one-and-a-half hours for just one night reduces daytime alertness by about one-third. Bottom line: without proper sleep, your body will not repair itself, you decrease the overall quality of your life, and you may even decrease your life span.

So, immediately after an acute injury, reduce the activity performed by that structure, do *not* perform weight-bearing exercises that can stress that area, do apply Cold Therapy, rest that structure, and keep it elevated to reduce inflammation.

By doing these simple steps, you provide your body with a critical element needed for self-healing...REST!

Exercise

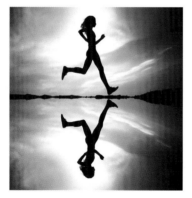

We have already talked about the importance of exercise in all aspects of your life.

When you have finished resting, icing, compressing, and elevating your injury, and once your inflammation has come down, you may want to start a moderate exercise program to get your damaged tissues back in gear.

This book, and its partners, show you how you can rehabilitate your tissues, and get back to an active lifestyle. Always start with the beginner's exercises to loosen those tight muscles and tissues, and as you progress, increase the intensity and type of exercise.

Remember, listen to your body...it is your best instructor and will tell you when you are overdoing things! So good luck...and get healthy and strong today!

Check our website at www.releaseyourbody.com for more information:

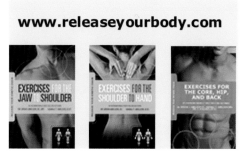

Release Your Kinetic Chain - Exercise Books

- Exercises for the Jaw to Shoulder
- Exercises for the Shoulder to Hand
- Exercises for the Back, Core, and Hip
- Exercises for the Hip to Toes

Release Your Pain – Resolving Repetitive Strain Injuries with Active Release Techniques

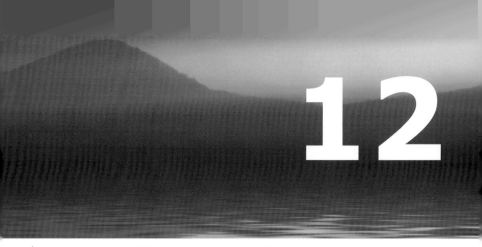

Alternative Therapies to Explore

The following section describes some of the types of practitioners with whom you might consider consulting when you have a soft-tissue injury that requires more assistance than exercise routines can provide. In all cases, to find the best practitioner, remember to check their certification and, where possible, ask for personal referrals.

Active Release Techniques® (ART)

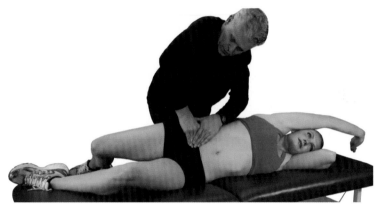

Dr. Abelson performing ART on the psoas.

Active Release Techniques (ART) is, in my opinion, one of the **most** effective and reliable methods for releasing adhesions or restrictions between soft tissue layers.

Just about any soft-tissue injury can be treated effectively with ART. This technique has helped Olympic athletes, PGA golfers, professional hockey players, and football players win numerous events. This multidisciplinary technique was developed by a Chiropractor, Dr. P. Michael Leahy of Colorado Springs, Colorado.

Essentially, ART is a hands-on soft-tissue technique that can simultaneously locate and break up scar tissue. The power of ART lies in how it combines patient motion with practitioner techniques to release the adhesions between tissue layers. This process restores mobility and relative motion to the soft tissue layers, increases circulatory function, and increases neurological function by breaking restrictive adhesions.

Effectiveness of Active Release Techniques

ART is at the top of my list for soft-tissue techniques, especially when it is performed correctly by a skilled practitioner. The key word is *skilled*! ART practitioners claim to have a 90% success rate, and this is quite true when the practitioner is both skilled and experienced. The key is to find someone with both the training and experience you require. As I mentioned, I strongly recommend Active Release Techniques® for the treatment and resolution of a broad range of soft-tissue injuries. But due to its growing popularity and effectiveness, there are many people claiming to be ART practitioners, who have **not** received the required training.

It is very important to check out the certification levels of your selected ART practitioner. ART practitioners can take courses in Upper Extremity, Lower Extremity, Spine, Long Nerve Entrapment, and Biomechanics. Make sure your practitioner is certified for treating the areas that you require. In addition (as one of the writers of the *ART Online Biomechanics Course*), I can tell you that it is well worth your time and health to find someone who is also certified in *both* biomechanics and ART. These specialized individuals will be better able to find and identify exactly which restrictions are inhibiting your performance, and then help you to eliminate the problem!

To verify your ART practitioner's qualifications, visit the Active Release website at **www.activerelease.com**. This site tracks all current ART practitioners, and provides information about their current level of certification.

Note: If you are searching by geographical area, you may need to click SEARCH several times, since this database will only display a limited number of doctors for each search. If you live in an area with many ART practitioners, the system may only display only ten at a time. So click several times to see all the ART practitioners in your area.

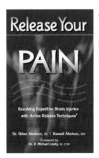

For more information about **Active Release Techniques**, you can also visit our websites at:

- www.activerelease.ca
- www.kinetichealth.ca.

In addition, to learn how ART can help resolve your soft tissue injury, you may want to read our best-selling book, **Release Your Pain** – *Resolving Repetitive Strain Injuries with Active Release Techniques*. Visit www.releaseyourbody.com for more details.

Graston Techniques®

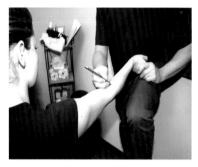

Graston Techniques® is an instrument-assisted, soft-tissue mobilization technique. The technique was initially designed by an athlete who suffered a debilitating knee injury.

Graston Techniques employs a combination of six hand-held, stainless steel instruments to release soft tissue restrictions.

The Graston instruments are used to separate and break down scar tissue (collagen cross-links). This process increases circulatory function and helps the practitioner to mobilize, reduce, and re-organize fibrotic restrictions in the neuromuscular-skeletal system.

As with other soft-tissue techniques, the practitioner must be skilled in the application and use of these instruments since considerable bruising can occur if this therapy is applied in too aggressive a manner.

The Graston tools can be of great benefit to many practitioners whose own joints and muscles suffer from Repetitive Strain Injuries (RSI). As a patient, this means your practitioner can use these tools to access severely restricted areas in your body, without causing further repetitive strain injuries to their own hands and body!

Graston Techniques® was first researched at Ball Memorial Hospital and Ball State University at Munci, Indiana. Today, there are more than 3000 clinicians—including Athletic Trainers, Chiropractors, Physiotherapists, and Occupational Therapists—who use Graston Techniques.

Effectiveness of Graston Techniques

In my opinion the power of this technique lies in its use as an adjunct – therapy, one which is best combined with other soft tissue modalities.

I believe this is especially true when the practitioner is dealing with nerve entrapment syndromes where he or she needs to find the location of the nerve, and release it from surrounding adhesed tissue, but must move through many layers of adhesed, entrapped soft tissue layers to do so.

Graston Techniques can be highly effective, especially when used in conjunction with other hands-on techniques such as Active Release Techniques, Manipulation, and Massage Therapy. However, after having applied both this and other soft-tissue techniques, I must say that there is nothing that matches the tactile sensitivity and effectiveness of a skilled practitioner's hands.

Note: With Graston Techniques it is common to experience some discomfort during the procedure, and find some minor bruising afterwards. This is usually nothing to worry about as it is just part of the normal healing process.

For more information, see www.grastontechnique.com.

Manipulation

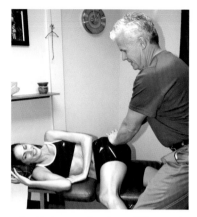

Dr. Abelson performing a Chiropractic manipulation.

Manipulation is used to treat musculoskeletal conditions, to relieve pain, and to improve neuromuscular function by restoring freedom to both spinal and peripheral joint movement.

In addition, through the effective manipulation of the spinal column and the body's extremities, there can be a substantial improvement in nervous system function.

Historical records show that manipulative therapies have existed for thousands of years. Manipulation has been documented in Chinese and Indian literature as far back as 2000 years ago. In China, manipulation has always been considered an effective form of therapy. This statement holds more weight when you consider that these Chinese physicians were only paid when their patients remained healthy. Now that is what I call a proactive health care system.

Today the most common types of western manipulation are Chiropractic and Osteopathic Manipulation. Both professions have a colourful history with no lack of controversy. The key point here is that all that controversy is historical! Today these medical professions are regulated by government bodies with strict criteria. Practitioners of both professions have no less than 7 years of post-secondary education. In fact, the first three years of their training is identical to any other medical professional.

Essentially, practitioners of manipulation move joints in a manner that frees up or breaks restrictions that are causing neurological or biomechanical problems. These biomechanical problems do not just include the joints themselves; manipulation also has a significant effect upon the body's soft tissues.

Manipulation affects muscles by causing the stress receptors in the muscles (Golgi tendons) to temporarily inhibit all activity in the areas being adjusted. This reaction causes the muscle group in the surrounding joints to go into an instantaneous state of relaxation. This intervention is a very important effect when your practitioner is trying to break a pain cycle. This approach to manipulation is strongly supported by scientific studies.

There are some opponents to manipulation that would still have the public believing that these therapies are unsupported. This is complete nonsense since there are literally hundreds of peer-reviewed scientific articles proving and supporting the benefits of manipulation.

Effectiveness of Manipulation

Manipulation is generally very safe and effective when performed by a trained professional. Just remember that manipulation can be used to treat musculoskeletal conditions, relieve pain, and improve function. I have seen hundreds of patient cases which would never have been resolved without manipulative treatments. On the other hand, for manipulation to remain effective, treatments must be combined with appropriate exercise. When manipulation is combined with soft-tissue techniques (such as Active Release Techniques, Graston Techniques, or Massage Therapy) it becomes even more effective since both joint and soft-tissue restrictions are removed or released.

Note: Unfortunately, some practitioners of manipulation get caught up in the marketing of their practices, rather than in achieving results. You may want to be a little concerned with practitioners who want to sign you up for a full year's worth of treatments!

Fortunately, this is not true for the majority of practitioners. The majority of practitioners are caring individuals who try to do the best they can for their patients. Good practitioners are going to try for the best resolution of your condition within the shortest time possible. The practitioner should provide you with a time frame for your treatment. For example, at our clinic this is usually 2 to 6 weeks (six weeks for severe cases). The practitioner should also provide you with specific exercises and other lifestyle recommendations that apply to your condition!

Massage Therapy

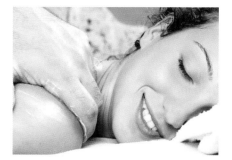

Massage is one of the oldest forms of touch-based healing. It can be used as a means of relaxation, or, in its deep-tissue form, to release restricted tissues.

Massage is not just an effective approach to pain management and rehabilitation, it also has tremendous physical, biochemical, and psychological benefits.

Massage increases circulatory function, increases blood oxygen levels, moves nutrients to needed areas, and displaces waste by-products. In fact, in terms of pain relief, some studies have shown that massage surpasses the effectiveness of numerous medications, without any of the negative side-effects.

Massage therapy has consistently been shown to help patients in dealing with their pain. This includes common muscle and joint pain as well as stress and pain arising from pregnancy, osteoarthritis, rheumatoid arthritis, and even cancer.

Massage therapy also provides huge psychological benefits in its ability to decrease stress and anxiety. Even stressed premature babies notice the difference. On the average, premature babies who receive regular massages gain 47% more weight than those who do not receive massage.

Effectiveness of Massage

Massage Therapy is very safe and highly recommended. Trained Registered Massage Therapists are very effective at treating and providing relief for a wide range of conditions such as migraine headaches, tendonitis, arthritis, osteoporosis, fibromyalgia, sports injuries, and a broad range of other common soft-tissue conditions. At Kinetic Health, we have several highly skilled therapists who work with us by combining their treatments with our own to help us achieve optimum patient results.

Finding a Massage Therapist

Since there are literally hundreds of different modalities that could be labeled as massage, there is no single governing body for the regulation of massage therapy. When you look for a Registered Massage Therapist, check for the following:

- Does the therapist have any experience in dealing with your particular type of soft-tissue injury?

- Does the Registered Massage Therapist have at least 1000 hours of training?

- How long has the Massage Therapist been practising?

- Is the Massage Therapist licensed?

- Who is the licensing authority and are they a reliable resource?

- Where did the Massage Therapist receive training?

- Does the Massage Therapist have any training in advanced or specific massage techniques?

- Can the therapist provide any supporting references?

Physiotherapy / Occupational Therapy

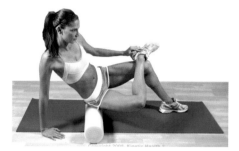 Physiotherapists and Occupational therapists are professionals who aim to rehabilitate and improve the condition of people who suffer from movement disorders.

To achieve their results, both professions use a combination of:

- Therapeutic exercises.
- Electrotherapeutic and mechanical agents such as ultrasound, TENS, short wave diathermy, interferential, ice, and heat.
- Functional training and some manipulation of joints and soft tissue.

Many of these therapists also take additional training in other techniques such as Acupuncture, IMS (Intermuscular Stimulation), Active Release Techniques, Graston Techniques, as well as a wide array of other procedures.

I teach courses with some great Physical and Occupational Therapists who I highly recommend. These individuals usually are very hands-on in their treatment approaches and provide their patients with individualized programs. They can truly be great resources of information. As a patient you could greatly benefit from this type of practitioner.

Effectiveness of Physiotherapy & Occupational Therapy

The effectiveness of Physiotherapy and Occupational Therapy, like many other professions, will vary greatly depending upon the practitioner's experience, skill, and the type of protocols that they implement. It is very important to find out from your potential therapist:

- What experience does the therapist have in treating your particular condition?
- How long will it take to resolve your condition?
- What type of results can you expect to receive from this treatment?
- Is the therapist licensed? With whom?
- Who is the Governing Body for this therapist?

It is also important to check on your therapist's current certification (via the local government body), especially where it applies to his or her additional training. For example, if a physiotherapist claims to be certified in acupuncture, check to see how much training they have actually received. Skilled Acupuncturists often have over 3000 hours of training, but many Physiotherapists (and Chiropractors) have less than 100 hours of training (not nearly enough, in my opinion).

You may also want to check if they are trained in areas such as Active Release Techniques or Graston Techniques. If yes, make sure their certification is current. When it comes to spinal manipulation, I would stick to a Chiropractor or Osteopath since a few weekend courses simply does not compare to four years of manipulative training.

Physiotherapists in Canada and the United States are required to register with a provincial or state governing body, with additional voluntary membership with a national association.

- If you are in Canada, visit **www.physiotherapy.com** for more information.
- If you are in the United States, visit **www.apta.org** for more information.
- For all other countries, please check with your state, provincial, or national organizations.

Acupuncture and Traditional Chinese Medicine

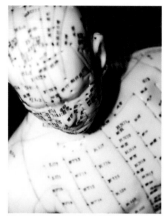

Acupuncture and Oriental Medicine are two of the fastest growing health care professions in North America.

Today, Doctoral training programs for Traditional Chinese Medicine (TCM) often provide an extensive curriculum which focuses upon both TCM and Western science. Performed correctly with great expertise, this can be a great tool for resolving many conditions.

For example, my younger sister, who suffered from partial paralysis after a stroke, regained full function within a short period of time due to treatments with acupuncture and oriental medicine. This is a great example how Chinese medicine can help resolve many conditions with which western medicine has had very limited success.

Western medicine is only just beginning to understand how these procedures actually work. Initially, many western doctors put the results down to the *placebo* effect. This attitude changed after studies by the Harvard Medical School using MRI brain imaging. Researchers using Functional Magnetic Resonance Imaging (fMRI) performed brain scans on normal subjects to investigate how Acupuncture affects brain activity.

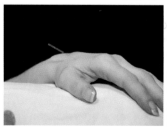

Acupuncture needle in the He Gu point.

All of the subjects had acupuncture needles inserted in the LI 4 (large intestine or He Gu point – located on the hand between the thumb and forefinger). In Acupuncture this point can be used to provide general pain relief during labour. Western medicine blew off this idea because there was no neurological or anatomical basis for this concept.

That was, of course, until they started testing the procedure with MRI brain mapping methodology. They found that the insertion and manipulation of the acupuncture needles at this point caused a pronounced calming of activity in many deep structures of the brain (amygdala, hippocampus, hypothalamus, etc.) accompanied by increased signal intensity in a key sensory region of the brain's cortex. There was only one conclusion that researchers could come to:

"Acupuncture regulates multiple physiological systems and achieves diverse therapeutic effects!"

Effectiveness of Acupuncture and Traditional Chinese Medicine

TCM can be very effective in the hands of a skilled practitioner. If you decide to seek out this treatment option, make sure you do your research and find out:

- Is your therapist certified in the technique?
- How many hours of training has he/she received?
- What experience does the therapist have in treating your particular condition?
- How long will it take to resolve your condition?
- What type of results can you expect to receive from this treatment?
- Is the therapist Board-certified and insured? With whom?
- Who is the Governing Body for this therapist? You should also be able to contact their local governing body to check on current certification.

As with all other Traditional Chinese Medicine techniques, these TCM procedures must be accompanied with appropriate exercise protocols. If a practitioner tells you that all you need is the TCM therapy and no exercise, then you should consider finding another practitioner.

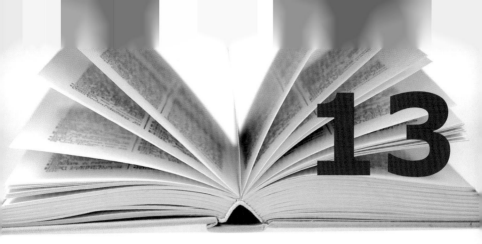

13

Index

Acknowledgements and Thanks

This book is dedicated to our parents, without whose support, inspiration, and love, we would not be who we are today! Thanks so much Mom and Dad - on both sides!

This book would not have come into existence without the participation of some wonderful people - our office staff, patients, family, and friends. We would like to take this opportunity to thank each and every one of you for your support and patience as we underwent the long, arduous, and sometimes frustrating process of writing this four-volume set of books! **Thank you, Thank you**, all of you! In particular, we would like to thank the following for their time, participation, and talent!

Our fantastic sports models - Jenny Fletcher, Arlynd Fletcher, Miki Waters, Sherry Sands, and Corrine Lloyd. Your knowledge, technical expertise, time, and friendship made these photos a pleasure to take, and a pleasure to use! You are beautiful - inside and out!

Our patient and thorough editors - Dr. Tarveen Ahluwalia, Hannah MacLeod, and Kristin Meidal. Wow, when my eyes got blurry, and my brain just couldn't process anymore, you were there to catch all those bugs, nits, commas, and funny little words I just couldn't see anymore! Thanks so much.

Our talented graphic artists - Our special thanks to Lavanya Balasubramanian for her superb illustrations and photography skills. You are without a doubt one of the most talented and artistic people in our life. Your grasp of our needs, and your ability to make our visions come true is phenomenal, and your sparkling energy and joy in life make you a delight to work with. Thanks also to Kirk Oulette for his beautiful cover designs and for bringing a fresh new look to our book covers.

Biographies

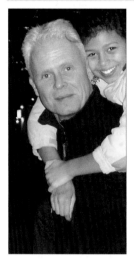

Dr. Brian Abelson DC - Brian's incredible, interdisciplinary knowledge of anatomy, physiology, human biomechanics, kinetic chain relationships, and exercise made these books possible. Just ask any of his patients, and they will fill your head with exclamations about how he can somehow *bring it all together* to solve their soft-tissue problems! And he brought it all together as we worked to design the exercise routines in these books...somehow integrating self-help exercises with his knowledge of soft-tissue restrictions, kinetic chains, and biomechanics to produce a graduated series of exercises that can help all of us to heal, recover, and perform at our best! Brian is a highly proficient Active Release Techniques Instructor and practitioner, trained in Graston Techniques, Chiropractic, Acupuncture and Chinese Medicine, Homeopathy, and Nutrition. He brings an integrated approach to health care which is very much appreciated by all his patients.

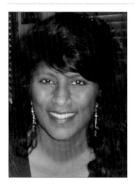

Kamali T. Abelson BSc - Kamali's long experience in the technical communication and publishing industry (25+ years) definitely came in handy as we wrote these books. Especially as they grew from the original vision of a 50-page booklet, into a four-volume set of books, each over 250 pages, packed with new illustrations, photos, and exercises. She enjoys the company of her friends, being a mom and wife, running, hiking, travelling, dancing, and the arts. Given the opportunity, she would be spending most of her time travelling to distant corners of the world, taking dance and art lessons, meeting new people, and absorbing new cultures, thoughts, and ways!

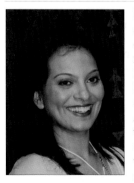

Dr. Tarveen Ahluwalia DC, BSc - Tarveen's medical and exercise knowledge combined with her friendship, enthusiastic participation, and technical edits helped to mold and develop these books. Tarveen is currently a Doctor of Chiropractic and Office Manager at Kinetic Health. She holds a Bachelor of Science in Kinesiology and is a certified Personal Trainer, and is a provider of Active Release and Graston Techniques. She enjoys time with her family and friends, speaking about health and fitness-related topics, and loves World music, weight training, running, hiking, travelling, cooking, reading, and Bhangra dancing.

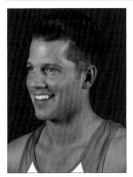

Arlynd Fletcher - Male model extraordinaire, with an amazing eye for positioning, light, and balancing photo shoots, all accompanied by a brilliant smile. Arlynd is also an incredible photographer in his own right! Brian and I bless the day we met you and Jenny.

Your help, professionalism, and ability to adjust the lighting to get just the right effect was priceless as we struggled to learn how to take exercise photos properly! You are awesome! Thanks so much for your help.

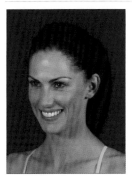

Jenny Fletcher - Supermodel Jenny Fletcher is incredibly photogenic and is also an amazing athlete. Every one of her exercise photos came out great. Today, Jenny is winning triathlons (*placing 1st in the 2009 Escape for Alcatraz*), appearing on the cover of sports magazines, and living an incredibly full life.

Read more about Jenny at www.jennyfletcher.com. It's been a privilege and pleasure watching you grow! Thanks so much for helping to make these books a reality.

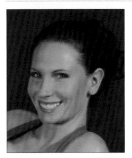

Miki Waters - Amazing massage therapist, great friend, and talented model...what more could you ask for! Oh yes...beautiful, too. Miki has been invaluable in getting our exercise vision onto paper. Her ability to hold a pose, even when the exercise leaves her quivering, is just another example of her professionalism...in all aspects of life!

Miki...it has been a pleasure working with you, getting to know you, and having you for a friend.

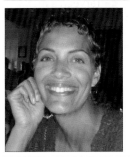

Sherry Sands - Massage therapist, wonderful friend, and a fountain of information. This multi-talented lady has been a part of our life for many years, and has modelled for both our international best-seller **Release Your Pain**, as well as other articles and publications.

She now works as a Production Accountant in the Calgary Oil Industry (did I say...multi-talented).

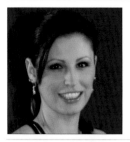

Corrine Lloyd - Another of our multi-talented, registered massage therapists, Corrine brought her brilliant smile, knowledge, and willingness to work hard at any exercise to all our photoshoots. Her joy in life brought exuberance and energy to all our sessions. You can see her in our books, brochures, and articles.

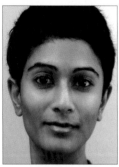

Lavanya Balasubramanian - This young lady brings sparkle and energy to our group...and never fails to lift our spirits. She is without a doubt one of the most talented artists we have ever met, and is able to take Brian's unique visions and present them artistically for our use, and your view. Her passion for our world, art, humanity, and the environment are a model for all of us! Here's to your continued growth...may you always sparkle bright!

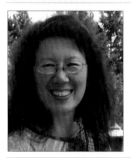

Hannah MacLeod - Wow...what a lady! Hannah has the most amazing eye for detail, and without her professional edits, and attention to all the details of presentation and content, this book would not be with you today. Of all our friends, Hannah has the most diverse set of hobbies and interests - from massage therapy and golfing, to knitting, spinning fibre, weaving, crafting, dancing, health, travel, and family! Love your YURTS, lady!

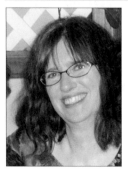

Kristin Meidal - Our long-time friend and co-worker. Kristin has a great eye for detail and pattern, and has helped throughout our writing process in ensuring consistency and clarity. Thanks again, Kris, for all that hard work; it's always a pleasure to work with you.

Publications from Kinetic Health

Written by the internationally best-selling authors of **Release Your Pain,** these books and exercise routines can help you release your pain, rehabilitate injuries, and help you achieve your best in both sports and daily life.

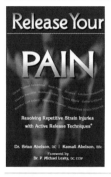

Release Your Pain - Resolving Repetitive Strain Injuries with Active Release Techniques
by Dr. Brian Abelson and Kamali T. Abelson

This international best seller has helped thousands of people resolve pain caused by repetitive strain and soft-tissue injuries, and is a great introduction to how the highly effective soft-tissue treatment method - Active Release Techniques - can help you recover from your soft-tissue injuries.
Available Now!

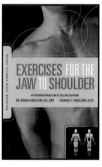

Exercises for the Jaw to Shoulder - Release Your Kinetic Chain by Dr. Brian Abelson and Kamali T. Abelson

If you suffer from headaches, jaw pain, TMJ, chronic neck pain, whiplash injuries, rotator cuff pain, shoulder pain, or other soft-tissue injuries of the jaw, neck, or shoulder, then this book may be exactly what you need. Instead of working with just the area of injury, these routines work with the Kinetic Chain, and can help you to take a key step towards resolving long-standing soft-tissue injuries and neuromuscular problems.
Available Now!

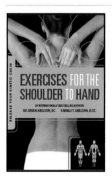

Exercises for the Shoulder to Hand - Release Your Kinetic Chain by Dr. Brian Abelson and Kamali T. Abelson

If you suffer from Shoulder Pain, Golfers Elbow, Tennis Elbow, Rotator Cuff Syndrome, carpal tunnel syndrome, wrist pain, or other hand injuries, this book reveals how everything you do – from working at your desk, to swinging a golf club - impacts the complex kinetic chain relationships within your soft tissue structures. The exercises are designed to help build and strengthen these neuromuscular relationships – a key step to resolving long-standing soft-tissue injuries, and improving strength, power, and sports performance.

Available Now!

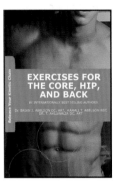

Kinetic Chain Exercises for Core, Hip, and Back - Release Your Kinetic Chain by Dr. Brian Abelson, Dr. Tarveen Ahluwalia, and Kamali T. Abelson

If you suffer from back pain, sciatica, or hip pain, have problems with core stability, or have the desire to improve your sports performance, then this is the book for you. Kinetic chain problems originating in the core are often the missing link for resolving chronic or acute injuries. This book takes you through a step-by-step process - from beginner to advanced - to release the power in your core and develop strength and flexibility without injury.

Coming Soon

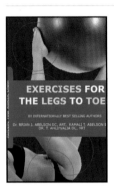

Kinetic Chain Exercise for the Hips to Toes - Release Your Kinetic Chain by Dr. Brian Abelson, Dr. Tarveen Ahluwalia, and Kamali T. Abelson

If you suffer from Plantar Fasciitis, Achilles Tendonitis, Iliotibial Band Syndrome, shin splints, knee pain, foot pain, or other lower extremity injuries then this book is for you. We considered key kinetic chain relationships in the development of each exercise routine in this book. Each routine helps strengthen key neuromuscular relationships – a key step in resolving long-standing soft-tissue injuries and in improving sports performance!

Coming Soon

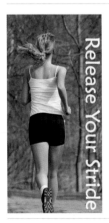

Release your Stride by Dr. Brian Abelson and Kamali T. Abelson

Runners, are you looking for a way to increase your running performance? Would you like to identify and correct those little biomechanical flaws that '*throw you off your stride*'?

This book gives you the tools you need to identify, correct, and resolve these problems, and get you performing at your best... whether you are a recreational runner or a professional athlete.

Coming Soon

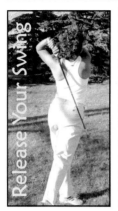

Release your Swing by Dr. Brian Abelson and Kamali T. Abelson

Golfers, are you still looking for that perfect club, the best ball, or incredible shoes, in order to achieve the perfect score in your golf game? Then stop for a minute! What may actually be stopping your game could be the restrictions in your body that prevent you from achieving that great golf swing.

Use this book to identify those biomechanical restrictions, and implement the tips and exercise routines to help release those restrictions, then watch how your kinetic chain gets activated to release your swing.

Coming Soon

Visit our website at www.releaseyourbody.com for more information and pick up your copy of these great books!